# Precision
# Livestock Farming

**NIPA® GENX ELECTRONIC RESOURCES & SOLUTIONS P. LTD.**
New Delhi-110 034

## About the Editors

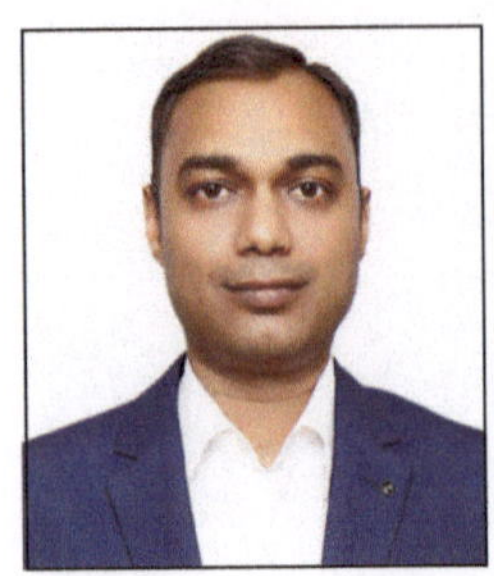

**Dr. Neeraj Kashyap** is currently working as Assistant Professor at the Department of Bioinformatics, and a faculty of Department of Animal Genetics and Breeding at Guru Angad Dev Veterinary and Animal Sciences University, Ludhiana (Punjab). He has done his masters from ICAR-Indian Veterinary Research Institute, Izatnagar and Ph.D. from ICAR-National Dairy Research Institute in Animal Genetics and Breeding. Dr Kashyap has a keen interest in quantitative genetics and molecular breeding of dairy animals. He has worked in various areas of dairy animal genetics and breeding such as heat tolerance, lactation curves, abnormal lactations and morphometry. He has been an Honorary Associate at University of Wisconsin- Madison (USA) in year 2023. He has also contributed towards applications of AI/ML and IoT towards catering the country specific needs of dairy sector. Dr. Kashyap has published over 35 research papers in journals of national and international repute and edited a book. His team has developed an IoT device for milk yield recording and trained ML models to record and predict milk yields of dairy animals from random test day milk yields.

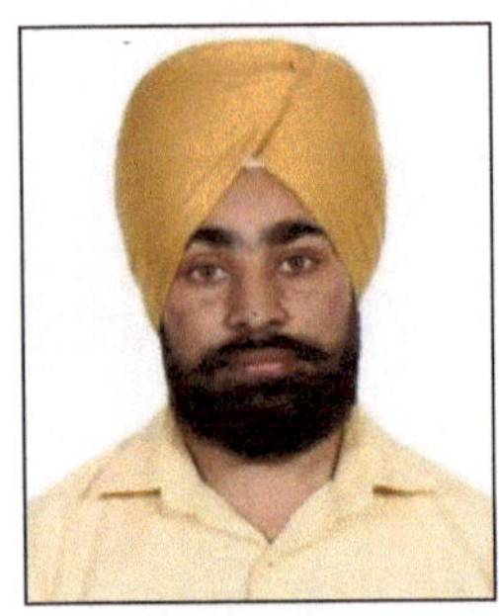

**Dr. Jaswinder Singh** is currently working as Professor in the Department of Veterinary & Animal Husbandry Extension Education, Guru Angad Dev Veterinary & Animal Sciences University, Ludhiana. During his 17 years of academic journey, Dr Singh Published 55 research articles in National and International Journals, 15 books, >300 extension articles, many leaflets/folders/calendars, delivered more than 400 expert lectures, attended two international training's, handled 8 projects, guided 8 PG students as major advisor. Dr Singh took many new initiatives to disseminate the scientific knowledge to end users. He started a digital newsletter for farmers, a YouTube channel, a Facebook page, a farmer portal and three mobile applications. He is also the editor of the University's monthly magazine. Dr. Singh has won the Best Extension Worker award from the institution twice. Aside from this Dr Singh has received others honours including Australia Award Fellowship, Associate Fellow NADS(I), Member NAVS and many more awards.

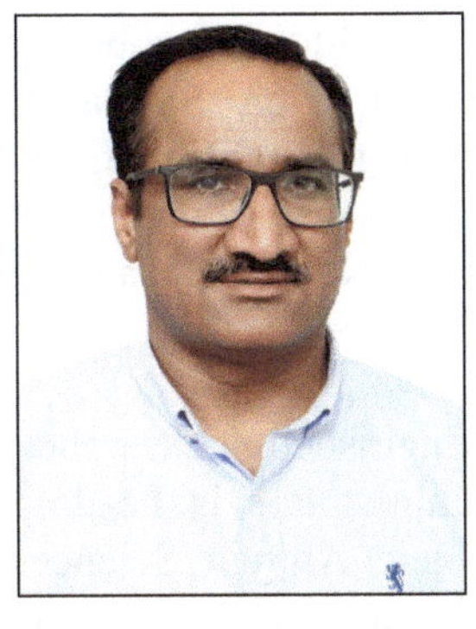

**Parvender Sheoran** is the Director, ICAR-Agricultural Technology Application Research Institute (ICAR-ATARI), Zone-I, Ludhiana, Punjab. He obtained his Ph.D. (Agronomy) from CCS Haryana Agricultural University, Hisar. His current areas of interest include developing location-specific best management practices (soil, water and crop) for sustainable crop production and exploring adaptation and mitigation strategies to enhance resource use efficiency in different agro-ecosystems. Endowed with outstanding academic and research contributions in the field of salinity management, oilseeds agronomy for more than 20 years, he has developed the agronomic package of 7 improved varieties/ hybrids of oilseeds crops (mustard, sunflower, linseed and sesame) released at National/State level, 22 farmers' worthy technological recommendations included in Package of Practices of Punjab/Haryana state, published 135+ research articles in high impact Journals of National/International repute, published 2 books, contributed several book chapters, success stories, technical/extension bulletins, extension articles, and delivered invited lectures, radio/TV talks etc. He has also developed a farmer's friendly mobile-app 'Salinity Expert' to aid the traditional extension methods in disseminating the salinity management technologies. He is recipient of ICAR-Swami Sahajanand Saraswati Outstanding Extension Scientist Award; Dr. PS Deshmukh Young Agronomist Award; University Gold Medal, ASPEE Gold, Australian Award Fellowship; AICRP-Rapeseed Mustard Team Award; CSSRI Best Scientist Award and Fellow of Indian Society of Weed Science and Oilseeds Research.

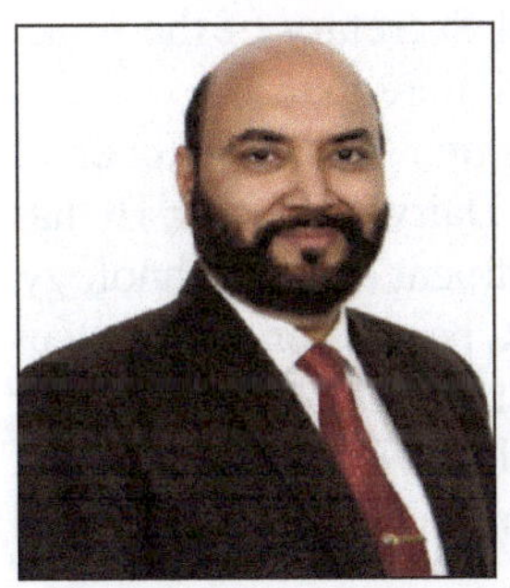

**Prof. Yashpal Singh Malik** is currently the Dean of the College of Animal Biotechnology, Guru Angad Dev Veterinary and Animal Sciences University, Ludhiana, India. He is a recipient of the prestigious position "ICAR National Fellow" at the ICAR-Indian Veterinary Research Institute. His areas of expertise are viral disease epidemiology, microbial biodiversity, host-virus interactions, and pathogen-diagnostics. He has pursued advanced studies in molecular virology at the University of Minnesota, USA; University of Ottawa, Ontario, Canada; and Wuhan Institute of Virology, Wuhan, China. He is the recipient of several prestigious national, state and academy awards and honors, including the ICAR-Jawaharlal Nehru Award. He has authored 9 books, 62 book chapters, and over 255 research and review articles. Prof Malik has been associated with societies of international repute, like, the Secretary General of the World Society for Virology (USA) and at national level serving as Secretary General of Indian Virological Society. Being a member in "One Health group in Federation of

Asian Veterinary Association" (FAVA) for 2021-2025, he is the Indian flag bearer on the international forum. Prof Malik is the Editor-in-Chief of the Journal of Immunology Immunopathology. His h-index is 56 with over 13000 citations. He has been awarded a prestigious Fellowship by the National Academy of Agricultural Sciences, Academy of Microbiological Sciences, National Academy of Veterinary Sciences and National Academy of Dairy Sciences.

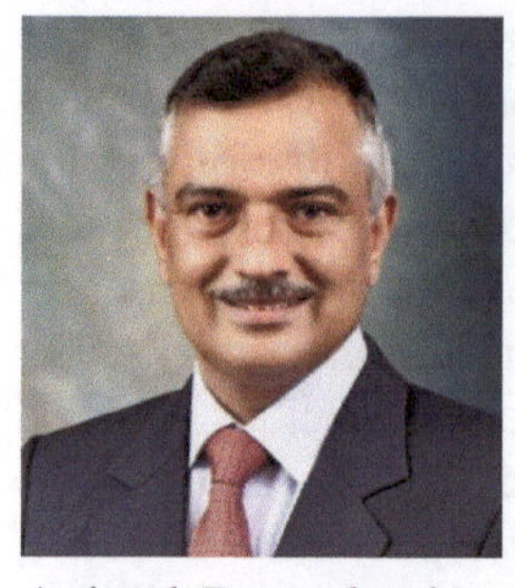

**Dr. Inderjeet Singh,** a distinguished researcher, academician and educational administrator is heading the Guru Angad Dev Veterinary and Animal Sciences University, Ludhiana as Vice-Chancellor since June 2020. Earlier, Dr. Singh worked as Director of Animal Husbandry Department, Punjab, for over one and a half years. He has a vast and dedicated experience of over three decades in the field of Veterinary Sciences and Animal Husbandry Sector. Dr. Singh did his Ph.D. in Animal Reproduction from University of Liverpool, United Kingdom. He has served as the Director of ICAR-Central Institute for Research on Buffaloes, Hisar (Haryana). Dr. Singh is Fellow of many scientific societies and has many feathers in his cap in form of scientific awards and recognition's. He is 'Executive Officer, Asia, International Buffalo Federation (IBF)', 'Member, Standing Committee, IBF', recipient of 'Distinguished Scientist Award by the Indian Society for Buffalo Development', 'Fellow National Academy of Veterinary Sciences', 'Fellow, National Academy of Dairy Sciences (India)' and 'Fellow of ISSAR', etc. He is the incumbent President of Indian Society for Buffalo Development. He has been the President, Vice-President as well as the General Secretary of the Asian Buffalo Association during various periods. He has visited more than 12 countries on various academic and research assignment(s). Dr. Singh is the member of National Advisory Committee for Animal Husbandry and Dairying Sector. He has served on various committees of the Govt. of India, Department of Biotechnology, Department of Animal Husbandry and Dairying and ICAR, besides on committees of Livestock Development Board(s) and Animal Husbandry Department(s) for implementation of central schemes and new initiatives like National Livestock Mission in the states of Madhya Pradesh, Andhra Pradesh, Rajasthan, Punjab and Haryana.

# Precision Livestock Farming


**Neeraj Kashyap**

Assistant Professor
Department of Bioinformatics
Department of Animal Genetics and Breeding
Guru Angad Dev Veterinary and Animal Sciences University
Ludhiana, Punjab

**Jaswinder Singh**

Professor
Department of Veterinary & Animal Husbandry Extension Education
Guru Angad Dev Veterinary & Animal Sciences University
Ludhiana, Punjab

**Parvender Sheoran**

Director
ICAR-Agricultural Technology Application Research Institute
(ICAR-ATARI), Zone-I
Ludhiana, Punjab

**Yashpal Singh Malik**

Joint Director, ICAR-Indian Veterinary Research Institute (ICAR-IVRI)
Mukteswar 263 138, Nainital, Uttarakhand
*Former* Dean
College of Animal Biotechnology
Guru Angad Dev Veterinary and Animal Sciences University
Ludhiana, Punjab

**Inderjeet Singh**

Vice-Chancellor
Guru Angad Dev Veterinary and Animal Sciences University
Ludhiana, Punjab

**NIPA® GENX ELECTRONIC RESOURCES & SOLUTIONS P. LTD.**
New Delhi-110 034

**NIPA• GENX ELECTRONIC**
**RESOURCES & SOLUTIONS P. LTD.**

101,103, Vikas Surya Plaza, CU Block
L.S.C.Market, Pitam Pura, New Delhi-110 034
Ph. +91 11 27341616, 27341717, 27341718
E-mail: newindiapublishingagency@gmail.com
www: www.nipabooks.com

***For customer assistance, please contact***
Phone: + 91-11-27 34 17 17
Fax: + 91-11-27 34 16 16
E-Mail: feedbacks@nipabooks.com



Print ISBN: 978-93-58875-87-4

ebook ISBN: 978-93-58874-21-1



Composed and Designed by NIPA®.

# Preface

Majority of the farming community are not aware of new developments that could help them with enhancing farm productivity, meeting their requirements, or solving problems. "Lab to Land" has become the motto for progression in agriculture and related sectors.

Disseminating the most recent research to end users involves the extension wing, a two-way bridge that connects researchers and farmers. It can do these organizing trainings, facilitating interactions between farmers and scientists, holding seminars and workshops, setting up field trips and camps, and utilising digital and social media platforms. If technology is confined to paper and within the walls of institutions, it is meaningless. Its full potential won't be achieved unless farmers—the end users,try it out in the field and provide input for further development.

Not every farmer in the region can be reached by the institute. For those farmers, district-level Krishi Vigyan Kendras, also known as farmers advising centres, are in operation. To meet the requirements of farmers in many sectors, these Kendras have a variety of subject matter experts, including specialists in animal science. These experts frequently collaborate with farmers at the local level and have the ability to ignite fresh ideas within the farming community.

In order to hone the skills and knowledge about the most recent advancements in the livestock sector. An interface between these extension workers and the scientific and academic community on "Precision Livestock Farming" was organised by the ATARI, zone I, Ludhiana on September 1-2, 2023, with technical support from the Guru Angad Dev Veterinary and Animal Sciences University Ludhiana.

Subject matter specialists and scientists working in different Krishi Vigyan Kendras (KVS) from the state of Punjab, Jammu and Kashmir, Ladakh, Himachal Pradesh and Uttarakhand attended the same along with few stakeholders as the representatives of the farmers communities.

To exchange knowledge, there were nine expert talks and a panel discussion. The technical lectures given in the interface are collected into a book format so that any subject matter expert working in the nation can easily refer to it.

Surely, this book will give the reader a new insight on the different livestock aspects.

**Editors**

# Contents

# 1

# Precision Livestock Farming The Concepts and Updates

***Neeraj Kashyap, Jaswinder Singh, Yashpal Singh Malik and Inderjeet Singh***

*Guru Angad Dev Veterinary and Animal Sciences University Ludhiana, Punjab*

## Abstract

*Coping up with the expanding demands for agricultural commodities along with ensuring the sustainability of production, requires a resource-efficient and more precise approach for crop and livestock management. The application of recent technologies as an integration of sensors, internet, cloud computing, robotics and artificial intelligence, has the potential to contribute to the cause, and when applied, they contribute towards data-driven decisions and automation in the farms and thus they are collectively called precision farming. The application of smart farming technologies is getting increasingly important in farming to assist in optimizing livestock production and minimizing waste and costs. Precision Livestock Farming (PLF) is a technology-backed approach to livestock farm management that records, quantifies, and infers the needs of individual animals and farms for optimal data-driven decisions. The present-day farmers need to use resources in a more optimized way to meet the growing demands for quality products and also to make the farming venture economically sustainable. To minimize the risks of livestock farming and maximize productivity, the PLF has currently evolved as a vastly researched and ever-advancing field. Thus, the PLF, employs the automatic monitoring of biological and behavioural traits of each animal individually, for keeping track of important animal and farm-related parameters viz. production, reproduction, growth and health along with the macro and micro environment, etc. To make the developed PLF systems accurate and commercially scalable, research is being conducted on the various steps and techniques involved in the development and operation of PLF applications, and thus the field is advancing at an astounding pace. The chapter here aims to give a brief overview of the concepts and updates on the recent scientific and technological tools in Precision Livestock Farming (PLF) and their applied contribution to livestock farming.*

**Keywords:** Precision Livestock Farming, Digital Farming, Data-Driven Decisions, Sensors, Robotics, Artificial Intelligence

Rearing animals has been amongst the most ancient professions of humanity and since the advent of domestication, the livestock keepers have been involved with them to a certain extent on financial, social and emotional fronts and thus have been curious about certain key aspects of the livestock under their care. The curiosity can be defined with the 'five W and one H' of questions as What needs to be done (requirements)? When to do that (timing)? Where are they (location)? Why is there a need (rationale)? How will that meet my purpose (state)? The farming community has traditionally been using these attributes for making farm decisions by observing the animals constantly, or periodically at key occasions such as milking. Such monitoring, aided by the wisdom of experience of the generations of farmers, led to the identification of the key events or problems in the health and productivity of individual animals. However, such kind of monitoring requires a deeper engagement in livestock keeping than that is desirable in commercial farming and the decisions/ detections are severely limited by the capability of the observer.

Precision Livestock Farming (PLF) is a term that encompasses the deployment of sensors for the capture of key biological information, the use of algorithms for processing the biological information (data science), systems for making inferences and making decisions based on the processed data (artificial intelligence), interfaces that allow for making use of these data (reporting) and implements for automation (robotics). PLF is intended to optimize the process of animal production, health care and welfare by generating vast real-time information to be used in various ways. There have been many systems being tried and found fit for practical applicability; whereas, few systems like geolocation and motion detection are extensively applied.

The potencies of PLF for livestock farming blooms through more objective and consistent capturing of animal-related information for increasing the efficiency of animal production, predicting risks to animal health and welfare, and determining animal status. Risks of increasing PLF usage include the dependency on technology and changes in the human–animal relationship. Veterinarians will be highly affected by PLF in their professional lives; nevertheless, they must adapt to this and play an active role in the further development of technology. It is much anticipated that PLF will bring a paradigm shift to the animal–human relationship and changes in the public perception of livestock farming.

The Food and Agriculture Organization of the United Nations (FAO) estimated that to meet out with the demands of rising human population, that is estimated to reach 9 billion by 2050, the food production also needs to increase by 70%. At the same time, due to economic growth of populace, the demand for quality food like milk, meat and other animal products is also rising. To ensure economic viability and improve profitability of the livestock keeping, the farmers are compelled to upscale their farms. Accordingly, the occurrence of farms with a larger number of raised heads, monitored by fewer farmers, is expected. Two additional important issues driving the implementation of modern livestock management practices are animal welfare and impact on environment. Hence, the automated real-time monitoring is progressively getting relied on in the livestock industry.

## High-Tech Herding for a Better Future

Precision Livestock Farming (PLF) is a way of using technology to manage livestock smarter, but not harder. It's like having a team of learned and skilled assistants monitoring farm animals consistently and providing insights, that one wouldn't get with traditional methods. PLF can be described as the technological system for real-time monitoring of farmed animals, aimed at managing the temporal variability of the smallest manageable production unit, known as the 'per animal approach'. The market for precision farming, including all sectors, is expected to grow at an annual rate of 13% to reach a volume of USD 12.9 billion in 2027, indicating that PLF is becoming ever more relevant for all aspects of livestock keeping.

As compared to the not so complex plants or microbes; animals, exhibit complex and individualistic behaviours which can vary from momentary response to lifetime habits. Such systems are referred to as "Complex, Individual and Time-variant" (CIT) systems. Thus, biological rhythms and behaviour involving animals have long been thought as too complicated to be monitored automatically and analysed in real-time. However, in recent two decades, new emerging technologies viz. sensors, algorithms, networking, are providing opportunities to develop fully automated online monitoring and control tools for many of these traits. Increasing the animal head counts and maintaining individual care to the animals simultaneously, has been a dilemma the farmers have faced for long. The concept of PLF was conceived as the solution to address the matter.

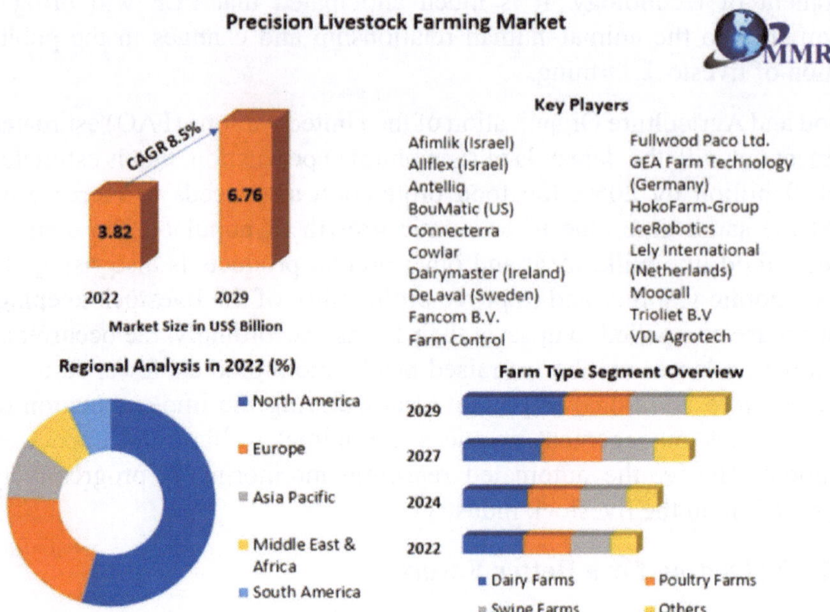


**Figure 1:** Dynamics of global PLF market (*Source*: https://shorturl.at/kCU17)

## Digitalization of Livestock Farms

In the context of livestock farming, the term digitalization may refer to sensor technology, electronic data processing and automated systems. Since the digitalization process of the livestock farms brings the advantage of timely and accurate reporting and alarms, the practice added the benefit of having precise information on the status of animals and farms; thereby raising the term Precision Livestock Farming (PLF).

PLF includes robots or sensors collecting and producing data which are computed and analysed by standardized operations (algorithms) to produce relevant information for the farmers, based on which the decisions for the farm would be taken more accurately. The algorithms analyze for traits of interest that serve as support or a basis for decision-making, mainly by the farmer himself. The key difference between PLF and traditional farming lies in rapid and accurate decision-making; facilitated by real-time capture of data, data integration from different sources, swift processing of data and the decision-making process, leading to in-time implementation of decisions. PLF, therefore, implies a system with implemented components like sensors, algorithms and interfaces for making practical use of data from livestock farming for the decision-making process.

The benefits that can be directly realized from the implementation of the PLF are:

- *Boosting animal health and welfare:* Early detection of problems means quicker treatment and happier animals.
- *Increasing productivity and efficiency:* Targeted interventions lead to better yields and resource use.
- *Improving sustainability:* Farm and animal data helps to optimize feed, water, and energy use, reducing environmental impact.

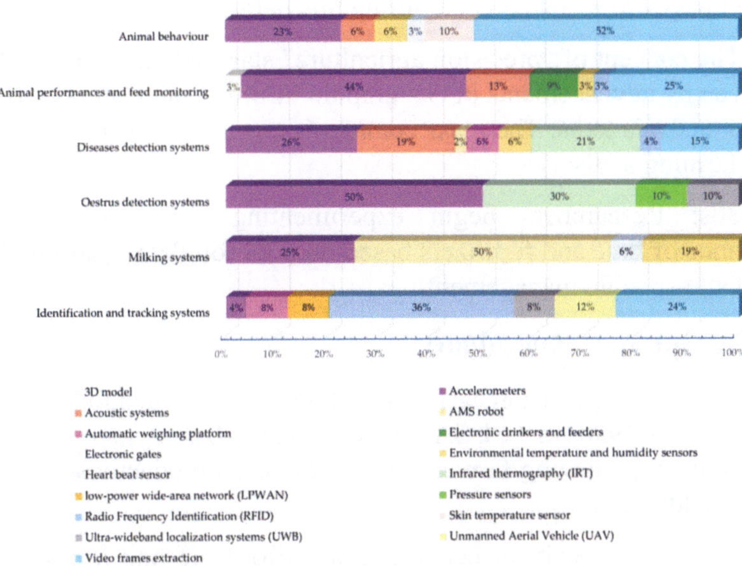


**Figure 2:** **Percentage of the most used sensors per each area of interest in PLF** (*Source*: Morrone et al., 2022)

While at present the PLF has its challenges in implementation, like cost and data security, the future looks bright for this technology due to its immense applicability. As it evolves, it has the potential to revolutionize animal agriculture, making it more productive, sustainable, and ethical. Overall, The PLF is a game-changer for farmers, enabling them to make data-driven decisions for precise actions based on real-time animal data; and implement personalized care leading to better outcomes and reduction in risks. The PLF also helps the farmers to work more efficiently by automating tasks and saving time, thereby the farmers can focus on strategic farm management.

## History of Precision Farming

The story of precision farming goes back further than one might surmise with its roots stretching back to the 1950s and it has started from the implementation of simple technologies, that might not be noticeable until pointed out. Here's a glimpse into its fascinating journey:

### Early seeds (1950s-1980s)

- 1950s-60s: The launch of GPS satellites laid the foundation for precise location tracking on farms. The meteorological forecasts based on satellite images were also crucial during this period.
- 1980s: The concept of "precision agriculture" starts taking shape in the US, driven by advancements in Geographic Information Systems (GIS) and data analysis tools. The mass communication media were used for issuing farming advisories.
- Mid-1980s: Researchers begin experimenting with variable-rate applications of lime and fertilizers based on field soil data, marking the onset of site-specific management.

### Growth and Adoption (1990s-2000s)

- 1990s: The idea of precision agriculture (PA) was presented for the first time in the early 1990s in the USA. Remote sensing-based yield monitors were developed, allowing farmers to measure crop productivity across different field zones.
- Late 1990s: GPS receivers become more affordable and accessible, paving the way for widespread adoption of precision farming practices. In 1997, the House of Representatives described PA as an "integrated information and production-based farming system designed to increase the efficiency, productivity and profitability of long-term, site-specific and entire farm production while minimizing impacts on wildlife and the environment".
- 2000s: The rise of the internet and agricultural software enables real-time data analysis and decision-making on farms.
- Precision agriculture expands from basic data collection to incorporating diverse technologies like crop sensors, drones, and robotics.

### The Present and Beyond (2010s-present)

- Focus on big data and analytics: Advanced computer models and machine learning algorithms helped derive deeper insights from farming data.
- Economization of technology: The advent of cloud computing mitigated the need for a local high-performing computer, the high-speed internet paved the way for efficient data transfer, and the availability of cheaper processors and sensors paved the way for developing affordable technologies to be applied in the farms.
- Integration with Internet of Things (IoT): Sensors embedded in farm equipment and infrastructure provide continuous data streams for comprehensive field monitoring.
- Rise of "smart farming" and "digital agriculture": Precision farming evolves into a broader movement encompassing connected technologies, data-driven decision support, and improved sustainability practices.
- Future trends: Continued advancements in artificial intelligence, robotics, and biotechnology are expected to further revolutionize precision farming, enabling even more precise and efficient management of agricultural operations.

### Key Figures

- Pierre Robert is often considered the "father of precision farming" for his early work promoting and organizing workshops on the concept.
- Researchers at the University of Minnesota played a significant role in developing the first variable-rate application techniques in the 1980s.

Overall, the history of precision farming reveals a constant push forward, using technology to gain a deeper understanding of individual fields and manage agricultural resources more effectively. As technology continues to evolve, this journey promises even more exciting innovations and a more sustainable future for agriculture.

## History of Precision Livestock Farming

Contrary to the belief, precision livestock farming aids are not the exclusive product of modern technology. Historically, one may find that innovative and applied techniques in their primitive form have been used traditionally by farmers. For example, a cow collar with a bell could be considered the traditional version of a remote animal monitoring device. The ringing of the bell enables a farmer to locate the animal and also gives insight into the status of the animal. The gentle ringing may denote a normally active animal resting or walking; whereas, a rapidly ringing bell indicates that the animal is running. The 'Industry 4.0' and 'Internet of Things' (IoT) played an integral part in the development and implementation of PLF. The IoT, conceptualized by Kevin Ashton in the year 1999, is a network of interconnected devices that communicate, sense, and interact with internal and external environments via embedded technology. The term Industry 4.0 originated in Germany in 2011 and has since rapidly been translated and adopted throughout the world. Specifically, this new paradigm is focused on automation, the incorporation of the Internet into industrial processes, and the dissemination of 'Information and Communication Technology' (ICT) to create intelligent devices, machines, and systems.

While precision agriculture has a longer history, precision livestock farming (PLF) is a relatively new field, with its emergence around the early 2000s. Here's a condensed timeline of its development:

**Early Stages (2000s)**

- Conceptualization: The term "precision livestock farming" was first coined in 2004, drawing inspiration from the success of precision agriculture. The first significant implementation of PLF was the use of individual electronic milk meter for dairy cows.
- Initial research: Pioneering studies focus on developing sensors and data collection methods for monitoring individual animals. The advent of wearable sensors led to the conceptualization of individual animal monitoring in real-time.
- Focus on dairy cattle: Early applications primarily target dairy farms, leveraging advancements in milk yield recording technologies.

**Expansion and Diversification (2010s onwards)**

- Industry 4.0: During the Industry 4.0 revolution, miniaturization and affordability of sensors led to wider adoption in various livestock sectors (poultry, pigs, etc.). RFID technology has played an important role in real-time animal identification and personalized data recording.
- Farm Automation: Robotics were used in animal management for automation of milking known as machine milking, automated gates were used for better herd segregation and management etc.

- Data analysis and modelling: Development of algorithms and software for interpreting animal data and providing actionable insights.
- Integration with other technologies: The present-day PLF is connected with robotics, cloud computing, and artificial intelligence, creating more sophisticated solutions.
- Growing focus on animal welfare: PLF applications increasingly address stress detection, disease prevention, and improved living conditions.

**Current state and prospects (2020 onwards)**

- Global awareness and adoption: The importance and applicability of PLF implements were acknowledged worldwide, for improving sustainability, animal welfare, and efficiency.
- Evolving applications: New technologies like image recognition and wearable sensors enable even more comprehensive animal monitoring.
- Integration with farm management systems: PLF data gets incorporated into broader farm management platforms for holistic decision-making. Now, a multitude of PLF techniques are integrated into a comprehensive farm management and monitoring system. One such system 'Dairy Brain 'was presented in 2020 by Cabrera et al. as an integrated system automatically optimizing group feeding and providing early recognition of cases of clinical mastitis. Thus, PLF appears to be developing away from only measuring parameters towards integration of different components and decision support or itself making decisions.

**Key Figures**

- Dr Janusz R. Wathes: A leading researcher in PLF, known for his contributions to behaviour-based monitoring and welfare assessment.
- EU Horizon 2020 projects: Several large-scale European research initiatives have significantly advanced PLF technologies and applications.

It is to be considered that PLF is still evolving, and its history is continuously being written. The future holds immense potential for this technology to transform animal agriculture towards a more precise, sustainable, and ethical future. The PLF has a lot of potential, yet there as certain challenges such as balancing cost-effectiveness, data privacy, and ethical considerations for wider adoption. This is particularly true for the farms in developing countries, where the average animal holding per farm is very small and the farms are scattered.

## Data-Driven Decision Making and PLF

Combining PLF (Precision Livestock Farming) with data-driven decision-making is a recipe for significant advancements in livestock farming. By transforming raw data into actionable insights, farmers can gain a deeper understanding of their animals, leading to improved animal welfare, increased productivity, and overall better farm management.

**It is very rational to use** real-time data on various parameters like vital signs, behaviour, feed intake, and environmental conditions **originating from PLF implements** make decisions beyond immediate farm management. The collected data is used for farm decisions such as alteration in feed formulation, culling/replacement/purchase decisions, breeding value estimation and selection and breeding plans. **Advanced analytics like** AI and machine learning can also be leveraged to analyse complex datasets, identify patterns, and generate actionable insights.

### Benefits of Data-Driven Decision Making

- **Personalized care:** Tailored management practices to individual animal needs, optimizing feed, water, and environmental conditions.
- **Animal Health and welfare:** Proactively identify stress and health issues based on changes in behaviour or vital signs, enabling timely interventions for improving herd health and welfare.
- **Animal Reproduction:** Accurate heat detection leading to improved conception, and calving alarms leading to reduced calf mortality are two major aspects where data-driven decisions play an important role, particularly by pinpointing the time for intervention.
- **Improved breeding:** Selection of breeding stock based on individual performance and genetic data accelerates genetic progress. Further, it is now possible to select difficult-to-measure traits like stress tolerance and behavioural traits due to the availability of data.
- **Resource optimization:** Reduction in waste and optimization of resource allocation by precisely matching feed, water, and energy needs and veterinary aid requirements.

### Challenges and Considerations

- **Data privacy and security:** Implementation of robust data security measures are required to protect animal and farm data from unauthorized access or misuse.

- **Data interpretation:** It is crucial to ensure that the farmers have the knowledge and skills to understand and interpret complex data insights effectively.
- **Algorithmic bias:** Training of AI models should be done with diverse data to avoid biased decision-making that could impact animal welfare or farm profitability.

The future holds immense potential for PLF and data-driven decision-making to revolutionize animal agriculture. Advancements in sensor technology, AI, and data analysis will continue to enhance data collection, analysis, and actionable insights. Collaboration between researchers, farmers, and technology developers is crucial to ensure responsible, ethical, and inclusive implementation of this transformative approach, leading to a more sustainable and productive future for the industry.

## The PLF Systems

### Components

The PLF systems have four broad functional components: (1) the device with sensor technology, which collects data; (2) the communication system, which transfers the data off the device; (3) the data handling and analytical system, which turns raw data into meaningful information; and (4) the data visualisation platform, which presents the information to the end user to enable decision making. The common sensors that detect the desired attribute include accelerometers, Global Navigation Satellite Systems (GNSS), proximity loggers, a power source that may include either an energy storage system or energy harvesting system or more commonly both; data storage and/or processing capability; and the packaging that contains all the elements, protect them from the external environment and attaches the entire system to the animal. Nowadays the most commonly used data visualisation platform is mobile apps and web apps that can be accessed from various handheld and computer devices.

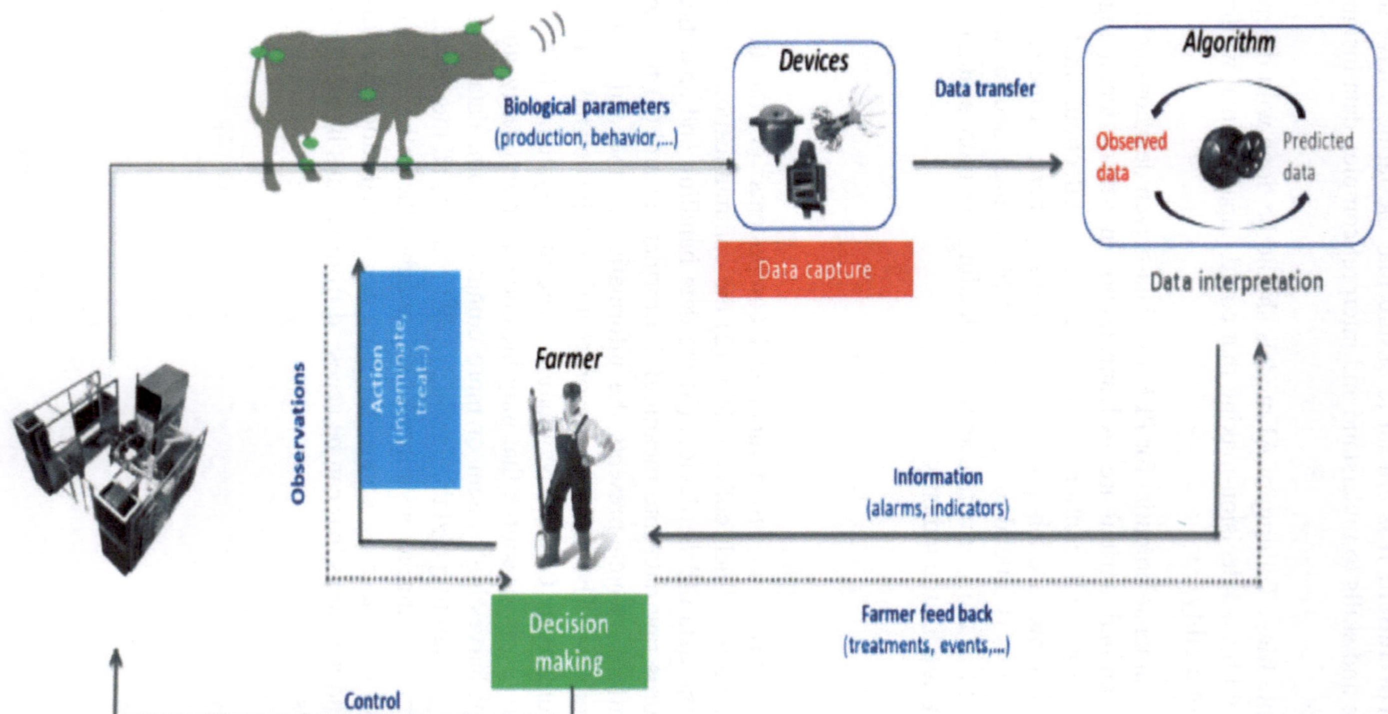


**Figure 3:** Overview of a PLF system of various components on a dairy farm (taken from Kleen & Guatteo, 2023)

*Sensors*: The Source of PLF Data

Sensors have been developed to record a variety of variables and come in diverse form factors, and sizes, and are capable of interaction with animals. Based on their site, the sensors can be broadly divided into two categories: off-animal sensors, which collect data by observing the animal without maintaining a permanent attachment; and on-animal sensors– which are attached to, or inserted into, the animal. Off-animal sensors include systems that automatically weigh, collect imagery or record vocalisations of livestock. Off-animal sensors provide valuable information, and a brief discussion of the benefits of integration between the two platforms is provided in the applications section.

Most of the on-animal and some of the off-animal imaging systems can monitor animals continuously on farms. However, on-animal sensors provide the convenience of being able to monitor each animal in wider and diverse conditions. The key advantage of on-animal sensors over off-animal sensors is that they collect information directly from wherever the animal is located, so the animal is monitored without being interrupted. This uninterrupted monitoring has grown as the key advantage of these systems, as such intense monitoring could never be achieved using farm personnel.

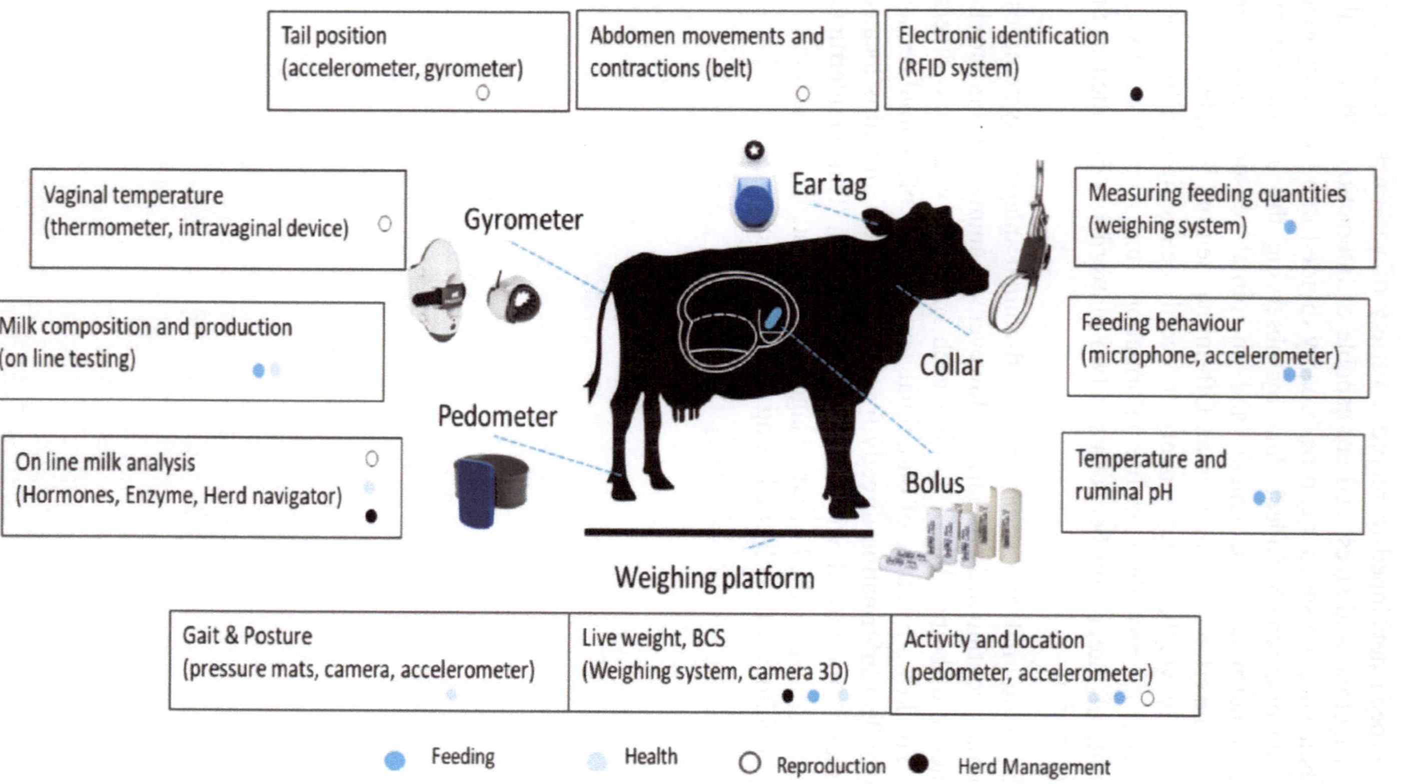


**Figure 4:** Overview of currently used devices to capture biological data from animals (Taken from Kleen & Guatteo, 2023)

## PLF and Animal Nutrition

Precision livestock farming (PLF) and animal nutrition are like a match made in heaven. By combining the real-time data from PLF technologies with the science of animal nutrition, farmers can achieve:

### Precision Feeding

Data on individual feed requirements, feed intake, behaviour, and performance; can be collected by the means of PLF implements, and that allows for calculations of customized diets that meet each animal's unique needs. Such individualized nutrition intends to optimise nutrient utilization and reduce feed waste. Monitoring feed intake patterns through smart feeders enables adjusting diets based on actual consumption, preventing underfeeding and overfeeding. Further, the PLF has automated the feed dispensing as per the nutrient requirement of animals.

**Targeted nutritional interventions** for animals with specific health concerns, are yet another field the PLF can help with Real-time adjustments in nutrients to address their unique requirements. Such as a high-yielder dairy animal can receive more concentrate in its feed.

### Improved Feed Efficiency

The individual feed consumption monitoring coupled with growth and production tracking can pinpoint animals with low feed conversion ratios, allowing for targeted interventions or culling decisions. Further, PLF sensors such as ruminal implants can track gut temperature and movement, providing insights into digestive health and allowing for adjustments to improve feed utilization.

### Enhanced Nutritional Welfare

Amongst the most successful dairy smart wearable technologies, the detection and logging of rumination patterns has gained prominence, due to its immense predictive potential. Changes in feeding and rumination behaviour often precede other disease and stress symptoms. PLF can detect these changes quickly, enabling early intervention and improved animal health.

Real-time monitoring of nutrient intake helps ensure animals receive all necessary nutrients, preventing deficiencies and related health problems. A further implementation is the use of precise feeding systems and optimized environments to mitigate competition and stress around feeding, improving animal welfare.

### Examples of PLF and Animal Nutrition in Action

- **Dairy cows:** Sensors track individual milk yield and feed intake, allowing for personalized diets that optimize milk production while minimizing feed costs.
- **Broiler chickens:** Image analysis systems monitor feeding behaviour and body weight, enabling adjustments to feed composition for faster growth and better meat quality.
- **Pigs:** Smart feeders track individual feed intake and activity, identifying animals with potential gut health issues, leading to targeted nutritional interventions.

Continued advancements in technology and research offer immense potential to create a more precise, efficient, and sustainable system for livestock nutrition, ensuring optimal animal growth and well-being while minimizing cost of feeding.

### PLF and Animal Health

Precision Livestock Farming (PLF) and animal health have formed a powerful partnership, transforming how farmers monitor and manage the well-being of their animals. Here's how PLF acts as a vigilant guardian for your herd:

### Early Disease Detection

The PLF implements provide real-time health monitoring by tracking vital signs like temperature, respiration, and activity, identifying subtle changes often preceding clinical symptoms. Further, the behavioural analysis is facilitated by cameras and image recognition systems, which detect abnormal behaviours like gait changes, reduced movement, or social withdrawal, indicating potential health issues. Integrating data from various sources allows for precision diagnostics, targeted interventions and early treatment, mitigating disease spread and improving recovery rates.

### Enhanced Disease Prevention

Environmental conditions are key factors in disease susceptibility. Environmental monitoring is facilitated by meteorological sensors that track temperature, humidity, and air quality, optimizing living conditions and reducing stress.

Preventive strategies like vaccinations and medication are also effectively utilized by identifying high-risk individuals, optimising resource allocation.

The biosecurity management is achieved by tracking animal movements and interactions helps isolate sick animals quickly and prevent the spread of disease within the herd.

### Improved Animal Welfare

The animal welfare can be improved by detecting and resolving stress and pain. Stressors like overcrowding or inadequate resources can be detected, allowing adjustments to improve animal comfort and reduce negative health impacts. Subtle signs of pain like difficulty in motion, reduced feed intake and isolation may be detected, enabling earlier intervention and improved pain management.

### Examples of PLF in Animal Health

- Detecting lameness in dairy cows through gait analysis, allowing for early intervention and preventing further injury.
- Detecting mastitis dairy cows through milk quality analysis and infrared image analysis, paving the path for early diagnosis and treatment.
- Identifying pigs with respiratory issues based on coughing sounds detected by microphones, enabling prompt treatment and isolation.
- Monitoring poultry flocks for signs of stress through thermal imaging, promoting adjustments to improve living conditions and reduce disease susceptibility.

The future of PLF and animal health holds immense promise. As technology advances and research progresses, this partnership has the potential to revolutionize animal welfare, disease management, and overall herd health, leading to a more sustainable and ethical approach to animal keeping.

### PLF and Animal Breeding

Animal breeding have a fascinating and complex relationship with the data originating from PLF practices, offering exciting possibilities of holistic identification of overall genetically superior animals, having merits in production, reproduction, fitness, confirmation, adaptability and tolerance to diseases. Now, it is possible to select and breed the animals for novel traits, those otherwise were too difficult to be recorded.

It is to be noted that, over-reliance on specific genetic lines for breeding could lead to reduction in genetic diversity in the livestock population, thereby increasing vulnerability to disease outbreaks and environmental changes.

Further, selective breeding for certain traits could have unintended negative consequences for animal welfare, such as compromising natural behaviours, pain perception, or overall health. One such occurrence was reduced adaptability among high yielding dairy animals for environmental stressors. Here are some key points to consider:

- **Enhanced selection:** By collecting individual data on performance, health, and behaviour, PLF can help pinpoint animals with desirable traits beyond just traditional measures like milk yield or growth rate. This is already leading to more accurate and efficient selection for complex traits like disease resistance, feed efficiency, and adaptability.
- **Precision breeding:** Combining individual animal data with genomic information allows for highly targeted breeding programs. Breeders can select animals based on both their phenotypes and their predicted offspring's potential, accelerating genetic progress toward desired traits. PLF in combination to genomic selection can identify promising breeding candidates at a younger age, reducing generation intervals and speeding up genetic progress. This is particularly beneficial for species with longer lifespans, like dairy cows.
- **Improved breeding management:** Real-time monitoring of factors like fertility and oestrus cycles is being used to optimize breeding timing and increase conception rates, leading to more efficient herd management.

## PLF and Genomics

Precision livestock farming (PLF) and genomics are becoming increasingly intertwined, creating a powerful duo for revolutionising animal and veterinary sciences. The techniques like GWAS and genomic selection require a large population for study that has been well recorded for traits of interest. The research experience has established that due to complex interactions between genes, environment and traits, a single gene or single trait approach often leads to ignorance of many possible causal relations. The data provided by PLF is as big and precise as genomic data and can thus be used for a wholesome genomic exploration of the traits.

## PLF Provides the Data

Sensors, cameras, and other PLF technologies continuously collect data on individual animals, their behaviour, health, and performance. This data paints a detailed picture of each animal's unique characteristics and response to its environment.

### Genomics Unlocks the Potential

By analysing an animal's genetic makeup, animal scientists can identify genes associated with desirable traits like disease resistance, feed efficiency, or milk production. By combining this genomic information with PLF data, farmers can gain deeper insights into individual animal potential and tailor selection, breeding and management strategies accordingly.

### Boost in Genetic Improvement

Selecting breeding stock based on both genotype and phenotype (PLF data) leads to faster genetic progress and improved herd performance, realizing personalized breeding. Integrating PLF data with genomic selection models facilitates more accurate predictions of breeding values, leading to faster genetic improvement and optimized herd composition.

### Examples of this Synergy in Action

- Identifying cows more likely to be high yielders based on genetics and proactivity monitoring and managing them through PLF implements.
- Breeding pigs for feed conversion efficiency based on their genetic information, real-time feed intake and growth data.
- Selecting breeding stock for poultry farms based on genes for disease resistance and PLF data on individual health status.

Integrating diverse data sources and developing robust genomic analysis tools remain ongoing challenges for integrating PLF data in genomics. The synergy of PLF and genomics together is already showing promising results as the animals are now also being selected for adaptability and behavioural traits. As technology advances and research progresses, this synergy has the potential to revolutionize selection and breeding, making it more productive, sustainable, and ethical.

### Future Technologies of PLF

The future of Precision Livestock Farming (PLF) is brimming with innovation, promising even more advanced technologies to transform animal agriculture. Here are some exciting possibilities on the horizon:

### Enhanced Sensing and Monitoring

Non-invasive wearable biosensors are being developed, to seamlessly monitor vital signs and internal health markers in real time, providing a deeper understanding of individual animal well-being. Advanced imaging technologies like infrared cameras, hyperspectral cameras and 3D imaging are able to capture subtle changes in behaviour, posture, or facial expressions, offering early insights into animal health and emotional state. The next level of monitoring achievable is an environmental monitoring at the micro level by sensors detecting minute changes in air quality, temperature, and even microbial communities within animal housing, enabling proactive adjustments for optimal living conditions.

## Artificial Intelligence and Machine Learning

The PLF is breaking from its shell of being decision support system to decision making system by implementing AI-powered decision support systems. Now machine learning is used to train AI for analysing vast datasets from diverse sources like sensors, genetics, and environmental data, providing farmers with real-time, actionable insights for personalized animal care and optimized farm management. Machine learning algorithms can more efficiently predict potential health issues, breeding outcomes, or even individual animal needs before they arise, allowing for preventive measures and proactive interventions. Such trained AI can constantly analyse data streams to identify unusual patterns that could indicate illness, stress, or other concerns, enabling early intervention and improved animal welfare.

## Robotics and Automation

Precision robotic feeders are now available those identify animals and on-spot formulate and dispense balanced feed rations to cater individual animal needs in real-time, optimizing nutrient intake and minimizing waste. Automated robotic milking systems with real-time milk quality monitoring are now being developed to not only collect milk but also analyse milk quality to infer udder health and early signs of mastitis, improving animal well-being and milk quality. Autonomous disinfection and cleaning robots are being deployed in the farms that can detect littering, automatically clean and disinfect surfaces and maintain optimal hygiene, thereby reducing disease risk and workload for farmers.

## Integration with Other Technologies

- **Blockchain for secure data management:** Imagine a secure blockchain network storing and managing animal data, ensuring transparency, traceability, and ethical use of information.

- **Internet of Things (IoT) for seamless connectivity:** Imagine all farm equipment and sensors seamlessly connected, creating a unified system for real-time data collection, analysis, and remote farm management.

## PLF in Developing Countries

Although, the Precision Livestock Farming (PLF) techniques have majorly developed to cater requirements of large farms as prevalent in developed countries, it also holds the potential to revolutionize animal agriculture in developing countries. In developing countries, where small-scale farmers often face challenges like limited resources, disease outbreaks, and low productivity, the PLF implements can provide exciting opportunities and can overcome hurdles:

### Opportunities

The potential for PLF to transform small-scale farming is undeniable. While challenges exist, ongoing advancements and targeted initiatives are making this technology increasingly accessible and beneficial for small farmers. PLF technologies can help small and marginal farmers optimize feed, water, and resource use, leading to higher yields and better animal health, ultimately improving income and livelihoods. Further, since majority of animal products are perishable commodities, PLF can help ensure quality of the products and prompt connection to marketing channels, by synchronizing the harvesting with market supply. Real-time monitoring through PLF can identify health issues early, preventing outbreaks and reducing livestock losses, a major concern for many small-scale farmers. By ensuring better animal health and traceability through PLF data, farmers can access premium markets demanding higher quality and ethical production standards.

### Challenges

- **Cost and affordability:** Initial investment in PLF technologies can be high, creating a barrier for resource-limited farmers. Innovative financing models and subsidies are needed for wider adoption.

- **Infrastructure and connectivity:** Lack of reliable internet access and electricity in rural areas can hinder the use of certain PLF technologies. Alternative solutions and offline data storage options need to be explored.

- **Technical expertise and training:** Farmers need training and support to understand and utilize PLF data effectively. Capacity-building programs and local support networks are crucial.

- **Cultural and social considerations:** PLF implementation needs to be sensitive to local cultural practices and social norms to ensure community acceptance and long-term sustainability.

**Examples and Initiatives**

- The **International Livestock Research Institute (ILRI)** is working on developing low-cost, accessible PLF solutions for smallholder farmers in Africa and Asia.
- The **Bill & Melinda Gates Foundation** is supporting projects that use PLF technologies to improve dairy production and smallholder livelihoods in East Africa.
- **NGOs** like Heifer International are training farmers in developing countries on basic PLF practices like using smart ear tags for temperature monitoring.
- The start-ups and major companies in developing countries are starting to develop locally relevant implements, such as Reliance Jio has taken initiative in livestock wearable technologies.
- Heifer International: Trains farmers in basic PLF practices like using smart ear tags for temperature monitoring.
- Precision Livestock Initiative (PLI): Works with partners globally to promote responsible and inclusive adoption of PLF for small-scale farmers.

Despite the challenges, the potential benefits of PLF for small-scale farmers and the growing focus on innovation and affordability make the future promising. Collaborative efforts involving researchers, development agencies, NGOs, and private companies are crucial to ensure responsible and inclusive implementation of PLF for a more sustainable and equitable future of animal agriculture in developing countries.

**Summary**

The PLF is possibly the most potent technologies amongst all the new and forthcoming technologies with the potential to transform the livestock farming. The aim of PLF has been to optimize farm management by streamlining animal production, breeding, nutrition, health and welfare. Further, since it is a rapidly evolving field, with only a few of the techniques being evaluated scientifically, it is early to fully judge and evaluate all developments. The possibilities for PLF to transform the way of livestock farming is vast. However, the research community and commercial technology developers need to concentrate their efforts on understanding what data and information are required by commercial producers to improve farm decision making and provide the benefits that these systems promise. The PLF industry has advanced in numerous ways since its conception in 2004, and this new generation PLF technologies are the key to further revolution in livestock keeping practices. With its ample present-day applications in dairy farms, the PLF has amply demonstrated its practical applicability and capabilities to combine sensors and information technology for animal behaviour monitoring, early recognition of stress/pain/disease, optimized feeding, precise management and improved animal welfare.

Yet, the alarms or reports on farm animals seem not to be the whole objective of PLF; rather, it is a comprehensive monitoring of the farm, and the whole industry. Rather than decision support, it is the smart decision making, is the real perception for PLF. As the available data swells in complexity and volume and gains accuracy, algorithms may be deployed to develop AI for automated decisions with immaculate accuracy. The data available may allow for a closer observation of farm events and development, better preparation of clinical activities or advice due to better data at hand and a more effective follow-up after changes have been implemented.

With increasing population pressure around the world and the need to increase agricultural production, there is a concern for improved management of the world's agricultural resources while minimizing the negative impact on the environment. The implementation of the PLF involves the integration of smart technologies in livestock keeping, allowing the farmer to manage farm variability to maximize the cost–benefit ratio and also to continuously and/or automatically monitor the main animal performance indicators. **Collaboration between researchers, development agencies, NGOs, and private companies** is crucial to address challenges and ensure responsible, inclusive implementation. Focusing on affordable technologies, capacity building, community engagement, and ethical data practices will unlock the full potential of PLF for a more sustainable and equitable future of small-scale agriculture.

## Suggested Readings

Berckmans, D. (2017). General introduction to precision livestock farming. Animal Frontiers, 7(1), 6-11.

Egon, K., & Oloyede, J. O. (2023). Advancements in Sensor Technologies for Precision Livestock Farming.

Kleen, J. L., & Guatteo, R. (2023). Precision Livestock Farming: What Does It Contain and What Are the Perspectives? Animals, 13(5), 779. https://doi.org/10.3390/ani13050779

Monteiro, A., Santos, S., & Gonçalves, P. (2021). Precision agriculture for crop and livestock farming—Brief review. Animals, 11(8), 2345. https://doi.org/10.3390/ani11082345

Morrone, S., Dimauro, C., Gambella, F., & Cappai, M. G. (2022). Industry 4.0 and precision livestock farming (PLF): an up to date overview across animal productions. Sensors, 22(12), 4319. https://doi.org/10.3390/s22124319

Zhang, M., Wang, X., Feng, H., Huang, Q., Xiao, X., & Zhang, X. (2021). Wearable Internet of Things enabled precision livestock farming in smart farms: A review of technical solutions for precise perception, biocompatibility, and sustainability monitoring. Journal of Cleaner Production, 312, 127712. https://doi.org/10.1016/j.jclepro.2021.127712

# 2

# Precision and Climate Change Livestock Production

***R S Grewal[1] and Inderpreet Kaur[2]***

*[1]Directorate of Livestock Farms*
*[2]Department of Dairy Economics and Business Management*
*Guru Angad Dev Veterinary and Animal Sciences University*
*Ludhiana, Punjab*

**Abstract**

*Livestock has been an integral part of rural livelihood and food security around the globe. Livestock as a vital source of food production utilizes vast amounts of resources (water, land, and feed) and has been linked with their contribution in climate change since decades. It is responsible for around 14.5% of global human-induced greenhouse gas emissions. Conversely, the effect of climate change adversely affects animal productivityand disrupts acid-base balance. With each unit increase above 72 THI the milk production decreases by 74 gm/d in buffaloes and with each unit increase above 70 THI the milk production decreases by 154 gm/d in crossbred HF. Also, feed intake in bovines declines with increase in temperature. There exists differences in the thermal tolerance between livestock species, therefore, there is need to select thermo-tolerant animals using genetic tools.Wind speed should be included in THI calculations for adequate measurements in climate change. Precision dairy farming tools viz., rumination and eating time sensors, activity meter, milking parlor-based sensor, body condition scoring camera, etc.should be implemented to integrate all systems on a single command computer. Nutritional corrections and management practices should be strengthened to check environmental stress on animals. To address climate change effectively, a comprehensive approach involving policy changes, technological innovation, improvements in animal efficiency, sustainable land-use patterns and shifts in consumption patterns is essential.*

**Keywords:** Climate change, Livestock farming, Precision dairy farming, THI

As per 20th Livestock Census (2019), Punjab has 1.3% share of India's total livestock. The share of buffaloes was largest (57.4%) in total livestock population, followed by cross-breed cattle and indigenous cattle. The state of Punjab has about 70.60 lakh livestock in total, comprising of 25.41 lakh cattle, 40.16 lakh buffaloes, 3.48 lakh goats, 0.85 lakh sheep, 0.53 lakh pigs, 0.15 lakh horses and ponies, 1644 mules, 471 donkeys and 170 camels. The share of crossbred cattle increased to 29.3% in 2019 compared to 25.4% in 2012 which signifies that the farmers in the state are resorting to high yielding animals for increasing the milk production. These efforts have led to the highest per capita availability of milk in Punjab which stands at 1271 grams per day compared to national average of 444 grams per day (2021-22), although the share of Punjab in country's milk production is 6.37%. Punjab is sixth largest producer of milk in India, with production of 14.76 million tonnes (t)/year.

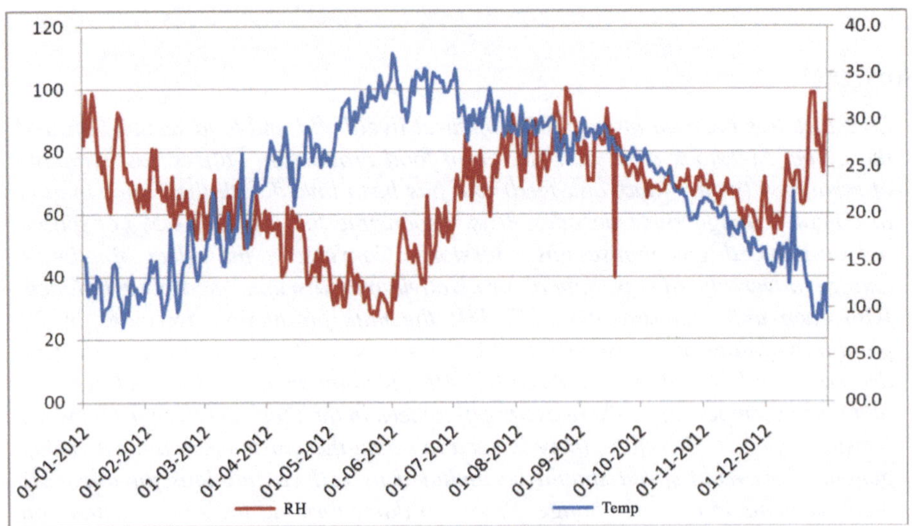


**Figure 1:** Monthly Temperature (Temp) and Relative Humidity (RH) in Ludhiana

Climate change has emerged as one of the most pressing global challenges of our time, with far-reaching consequences for ecosystems, economies, and societies. This has led to the higher temperatures, changing precipitation patterns, sea level rise and growing frequency and intensity of extreme weather events such as drought, floods, extreme heat and cyclones resulting in disruption of food supply chains. The most critical domains that impact environmental sustainability includes energy, transport, food, waste and water , although there are disparities in the consumption patten of high-income and low-income countries. Apart from the food domain (33% of total GHG emissions), meat from ruminants and dairy products constitute the major proportion of carbon footprint. Although only 18% of calories are obtained from meat and dairy products, but they together account for 60% of agriculture's greenhouse gas emissions and occupy 83% of the world's arable land. With 18% of anthropogenic greenhouse gas (GHG) emissions, the livestock sector has been identified as one of the primary causes of climate change and the dairysector accounts for around 3.0- 5.1% of the total GHG emissions globally.

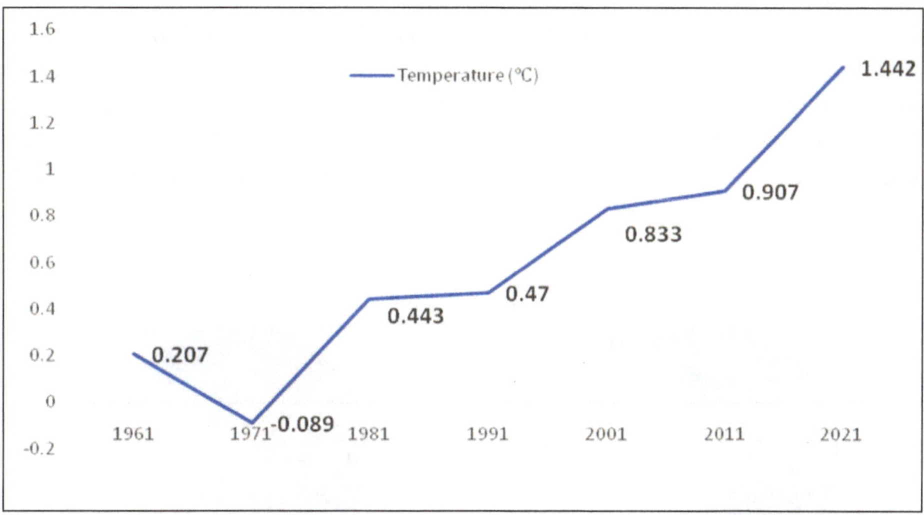


**Figure 2:** Temperature change *w.r.t.* a baseline climatology, corresponding to the period 1951–1980. (*Source:* FAOSTAT, 2021)

Livestock production, while essential for food security and livelihoods, is associated with significant environmental implications, particularly in relation to greenhouse gas emissions, deforestation, and resource consumption. In this context, livestock sector is considered as one of the important domains to achieve the United Nation Sustainable Development Group (UNSDG) 2030 to limit the temperature below 1.5C as per the Paris Agreement on Climate Change. In the backdrops of these environmental concerns and target to reach the net zero carbon emissions by 2050, it is crucial to delve into the intricate relationship between livestock and climate change, highlighting the key factors contributing to their interconnection and potential strategies to mitigate their impact.

## Livestock's Carbon Footprint

The total livestock population has increased by 27.34% from 1997 to 2019 with increase in total bovine population by 17.8% in the same period. Livestock farming is a substantial source of greenhouse gas emissions, particularly methane ($CH_4$) and nitrous oxide ($N_2O$). These gases are significantly more potent in terms of their heat-trapping ability than carbon dioxide ($CO_2$), albeit present in smaller quantities. Methane is produced during enteric fermentation in the stomachs of ruminant animals like cattle, sheep, and goats, as well as during manure decomposition. Nitrous oxide, on the other hand, is released from manure management and the use of synthetic fertilizers in feed production. According to the Food and Agriculture Organization (FAO), livestock production is responsible for nearly 14.5% of global human-induced greenhouse gas emissions. Cattle, particularly beef cattle, are the largest contributors due to their extensive land requirements, methane emissions, and energy-intensive production processes. Thus, efforts to address climate change must include a critical examination of livestock agriculture's carbon footprint.

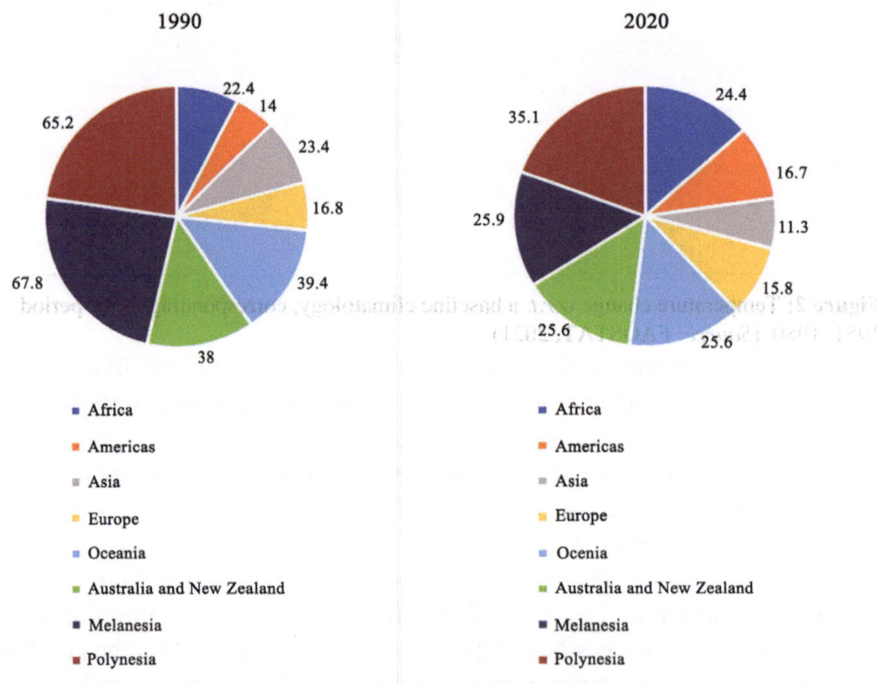


**Figure 3:** Percentage (%) share of farm gate emissions ($CO_2$eq) in various continents (*Source*: FAOSTAT, 2022)

## Resource Intensiveness

The expansion of livestock agriculture often drives deforestation and land-use change, which exacerbate climate change. Forests act as carbon sinks, absorbing $CO_2$ from the atmosphere, but when trees are cleared for pasture or feed production, this carbon storage is lost. Moreover, the conversion of forests to pasture or cropland can disrupt local ecosystems, leading to biodiversity loss and altering regional weather patterns. In the Amazon rainforest, for instance, large areas have been cleared to make way for cattle ranching. This not only releases stored carbon into the atmosphere but also reduces the forest's capacity to act as a buffer against climate change impacts. Sustainable land-use practices that minimize deforestation and promote reforestation are crucial components of mitigating the effects of livestock on climate change.

Livestock production requires vast amounts of resources, including water, land, and feed. Inefficient feed conversion rates, where a significant portion of crops grown for animal feed is lost in the process, contribute to the resource-intensiveness of livestock agriculture. This puts pressure on water supplies and exacerbates competition for arable land. Furthermore, the production of feed crops often involves the use of synthetic fertilizers, which release nitrous oxide into the atmosphere. These fertilizers not only contribute to greenhouse gas emissions but can also lead to nutrient runoff, causing water pollution and ecosystem degradation.

## Climate and Bovine Performance in India

Heat stress is defined as the sum of external forces acting on an animal that causes an increase in body temperature and evokes a physiological response. Excessive heat load on animal can lead to disturbed physiological functions and reduced performance. Documented physiological coping strategies used by dairy cows include increased respiration rate, panting, and sweating, and reduced milk yield and reproductive performance. Feed intake reduces more rapidly above 30°C in temperate climatic condition and at 40°C it may decline by as much as 40%. There is huge economic loss due to heat stress in livestock. In India, there is loss of 1.8 million tonnes of milk a year due to heat stress among cattle and buffaloes, which is attributable to approximately Rs. 2661 crore.

Heat stress is generally parameterised by the Temperature-Humidity Index, which combines ambient temperature and relative humidity to express an indicator of the degree of heat stress.

## Milk Production and Composition

Heat Stress (HS) adversely affects milk production and its composition in dairy animals, especially high milk producing animals. In response to heat stress the dairy cows reduce feed intake which is directly associated with

Negative Energy Balance (NEB), which is responsible for the decline in milk production. Drop in milk production up to 50% in dairy animals might be due to reduced feed intake, rest could be reasons of metabolic adaptations to HS as HS response markedly alters post-absorptive carbohydrate, lipid, and protein metabolism a part of reduced feed intake.

The stage of lactation is an important factor for severity of imposed HS and animals which in mid-lactation are mostly heat sensitive compared to early and late. Continual genetic selection of dairy animals for greater performance results to increased HS sensitivity and decreasing trend in lactation curve with poor milk quality in summer seasons.

**Milk production decrease in buffaloes:** Regression model fitted for decline in daily milk yield beyond Trigger Point of THI

- Regression Coefficient (β) = -0.0724±0.0018
- Decline in daily milk yield for per unit increase in THI
- Model fitted with an R square value of 0.634
- Lower Limit of rate of decline in daily milk yield
- $(\beta+SE_\beta)$ = 0.071 litres per unit THI increase
- **Upper limit of rate of decline in daily milk yield**
- **$(\beta-SE_\beta)$ = 0.074 litres per unit THI increase**

With each unit increase above 72THI the milk production decreases by 74 gm/d in buffaloes.

**Milk production decrease in crossbred cows:** Regression model fitted for decline in daily milk yield beyond Trigger Point of THI

- Regression Coefficient (β) = -0.1494±0.0045
- Decline in daily milk yield for per unit increase in THI
- Model fitted with an R square value of 0.572
- Lower Limit of rate of decline in daily milk yield
- $(\beta+SE_\beta)$ = 0.145 litres per unit THI increase
- **Upper limit of rate of decline in daily milk yield**
- **$(\beta-SE_\beta)$ = 0.154 litres per unit THI increase**

With each unit increase above 70 THI the milk production decreases by 154 gm/d in crossbred HF.

## Heat Stress Management

The environmental conditions driving heat stress are presented using the unit less temperature-humidity index **(THI),** a calculated index that incorporates the effects of environmental temperature with relative humidity. THI <71 as a thermal comfort zone (assuming the THI does not drop below the thermoneutral conditions of dairy cows, which induces cold stress), 72 to 79 as mild heat stress, 80 to 90 as moderate heat stress, and >90 as severe heat stress.On the basis of THI, three different zones as non-heat stress zone (NHSZ), heat stress zone (HSZ) and critical heat stress zone (CHSZ) has been identified. The months from October to March were included under NHSZ with THI values 56.71-73.21 and months from April to September were incorporated under HSZ with THI values 75.39-81.60 while the months of May and June were identified as the CHSZ within the HSZ with THI values 80.27-81.60. However, the categorical THI values can only act as a rough indicator for the effects of heat stress on production measures, in lieu of knowing the animal's internal body temperature. Wind speed has also been shown to affect environmental temperatures and should be included in THI calculations when possible.

Clearly, with nutritional corrections and management practices, the effect of heat stress on dairy animals can be alleviated. Therefore, in order to prevent the effects of heat stress, the modification of the surrounding environment is the key management practices to be followed in the dairy herd. Primary methods for altering the environment can be classified into two categories; first is the provision of shade and the other is evaporative cooling strategies with water. Theoretically, ideal type of animal shelters should maintain micro environment temperature between 15 to 25°C and humidity level around 10-12 mm Hg. The long axis of the shed should be in east-west direction. This east-west orientation helps to keep the shelter shaded for most of the day. Open type of shed is preferred in hot dry and hot humid climate.

Various cooling options for dairy cows exist based on the principles of convection, conduction, radiation, and evaporation. Though the evaporative cooling strategies are costly, but they are more useful to alleviate the heat stress in animals. Evaporative cooling systems use the energy from the air to evaporate water and evaporation of water into warm air reduces the air temperature. The milk production and reproductive performances of dairy cattle were improved using an evaporative cooling system. Fogging systems use very fine droplets of water and these water droplets are immediately dispersed into the air stream and quickly evaporate, thus cooling the surrounding air. Misting systems generate larger droplets than fogging systems, but cool the air by the same principle. The sprinklers are different from forgers and misters. The sprinklers do not cool the air rather than the large droplet arising from them wet the hair coat and skin of the cows and buffaloes and then water evaporates to cool the hair and skin. This system is a very effective in combination with air movement. The mechanical air cooling is possible by using the evaporative cooling pad and fan system which are very useful in reducing the rectal temperature and respiratory rate in cows and buffaloes. Sprinkler-system water use can range from 215 L/cow per day to 454.2 L/cow per day, quantities that may become economically and environmentally unsustainable in the near future.

However, long-term strategies have to be evolved for adaptation to climate change. Differences in thermal tolerance exist between livestock species provide tools to select thermo-tolerant animals using genetic tools. The identification of heat-tolerant animals within high-producing breeds will be useful only if these animals are able to maintain high productivity and survivability when exposed to heat stress conditions. Cattle with shorter hair, hair of greater diameter and lighter coat color are more adapted to hot environments than those with longer hair coats and darker colors.

## Dry Matter Intake

The increase in environmental temperature has a direct negative effect on appetite center of the hypothalamus to decreases feed intake. Feed intake declines at temperatures of 25-26°C in lactating HF cows and reduces more sharply above 30°C in and at 40°C it may decline by as much as 40% and8-10% in buffalo heifers. Due to this the animal experience a negative energy balance (NEB), resulting in decrease in body weight and body condition score. There are reports that indicate that under heat stress the acetate production in rumen reduces and propionate and butyrate production increases. Due to this animal reduces intake and rumen pH also decreases and ranges from 5.82 to 6.03. This adversely affects the rumen motility and rumination. Impairment of thyroid function can also be observed.

## Acid-base Balance

During heat stress animal losses more fluid by respiration and sweating that increases the maintenance requirements to control dehydration and blood homeostasis. Increase in respiration rate results in more loss of $CO_2$ which decreases carbonic acid in blood leading to increased bicarbonate and blood alkalosis. Animal excrete bicarbonate through urine to maintain carbonic acid-bicarbonate ratio. Prolonged hyperthermia leads to severe depression in dry matter intake which leads to prolonged ruminal acidosis.

## Precision Dairy Farming

Precision Dairy Farming is the use of technologies to measure physiological, behavioural, and production indicators on individual animals to improve management strategies and farm performance. With increase in herd size the use of sensor based tools for farm management becomes very important. Most of the time these are single unit put on animal as neck collars which also give animal ID and other information through antenna to computer. The computer is attached with milking parlor which gives milk yield directly into computer. Some of tools are as follows:

***Rumination and eating time sensors*:** These are neck collar-based sensor which measures the rumination time and eating time and correlate it to health of animals

***Activity meter:*** These are either integrated in neck collars or attached as separate sensor on hind leg. These are very useful in giving indication for estrus of animal.

***Milking parlor-based sensor*:** Advanced sensor like for measuring milk conductivity, SCC and milk composition are also attached with milking parlor.

***Body condition scoring camera:*** This is installed near milking parlor, which is integrated with neck collar animal ID and it gives animal BCS directly to computer.

These tools of precision dairy farming should be implemented in well thought out manner so that all systems can be integrated on a single command computer.

## Mitigation Strategies

Addressing the impact of livestock on climate change requires a multi-faceted approach involving stakeholders from governments, industries, and consumers. Some potential strategies include:

1. ***Efficiency Improvements**:* Implementing practices that improve livestock productivity, such as better animal genetics, efficient feed management, and waste reduction, can reduce emissions per unit of output.
2. ***Shift in Diets**:* Encouraging a shift towards plant-based diets or alternatives to meat can significantly reduce the demand for livestock products and subsequently decrease the pressure on resources and emissions.

3. ***Sustainable Land Use:*** Enforcing policies that discourage deforestation and promote sustainable land-use practices can help preserve carbon sinks and maintain ecosystem services.
4. ***Manure Management:*** Implementing improved manure management techniques, such as anaerobic digestion, can capture methane emissions and convert them into biogas for energy production.
5. **Technological Innovation:** Investing in research and development of technologies like livestock feed additives that reduce methane emissions or carbon capture and storage techniques can provide innovative solutions.

## Conclusion

The nexus between livestock production and climate change is complex and multifaceted. While livestock agriculture plays a vital role in food security and livelihoods, its environmental impact, particularly in terms of greenhouse gas emissions, deforestation, and resource consumption, cannot be ignored. To address climate change effectively, a comprehensive approach involving policy changes, technological innovation, and shifts in consumption patterns is essential. Balancing the need for sustainable food production with the imperative to mitigate climate change requires collective action and a commitment to a more environmentally conscious future.

## Suggested Readings

Dash, S., Chakravarty, A. K., Singh, A., Behera, R., Upadhyay, A., &Shivahre, P. R. (2014). Determination of critical heat stress zone for fertility traits using temperature humidity index in Murrah buffaloes. Indian J. Anim. Sci, 84(11), 1181-1184.

Halachmi, I. (Ed.). (2015). Precision livestock farming applications: Making sense of sensors to support farm management. Wageningen Academic Publishers.

Koltes, J. E., Koltes, D. A., Mote, B. E., Tucker, J., & Hubbell III, D. S. (2018). Automated collection of heat stress data in livestock: new technologies and opportunities. Translational Animal Science, 2(3), 319-323.

Lovarelli, D., Bacenetti, J., &Guarino, M. (2020). A review on dairy cattle farming: Is precision livestock farming the compromise for an environmental, economic and social sustainable production?. Journal of Cleaner Production, 262, 121409.

Patra, A. K. (2017). Accounting methane and nitrous oxide emissions, and carbon footprints of livestock food products in different states of India. Journal of Cleaner Production, 162, 678-686.

Pelletier, N., &Tyedmers, P. (2010).Forecasting potential global environmental costs of livestock production 2000–2050. Proceedings of the National Academy of Sciences, 107(43), 18371-18374.

# 3

# Use of Crop Residues as Alternative Feed Ingredients in Animal Feeding

***Shasta Kalra, Jaspal Singh Hundal and Jaswinder Singh***

*Department of Animal Nutrition, Guru Angad Dev Veterinary and Animal Sciences University, Ludhiana, Punjab*

**Abstract**

*The intensive livestock production continues to face challenges and limitations due to the increasing cost of fossil fuels, competition for food-feed fuel, and other biophysical limiting factors, challenging the sustainability of the animal production systems. A shortage of feed and fodder in India and other parts of the world has led to an increased interest in utilizing agricultural by-products such as crop residues as alternative feed ingredients for livestock. Terrestrial animals, especially ruminants, are characterized by their ability to convert low-quality roughage into high-value products, e.g., meat, milk, natural fibers, leather, and manure. These by-products constitute an important and often the major feed resource available, and their utilization is growing because of the ever-decreasing access to free grazing areas as well as the increase in the cost of commercial feed. Therefore, having appropriate information on the quality and quantity of these feedstuffs helps to fulfill the dietary requirements of the animals at relatively lower expenses. The techniques of feeding these residues range from traditional stubble-grazing of harvested grain fields to the preparation of chopped residue mixes based on a total mixed ration and ensilage that are made more palatable and nutritious by the addition of nutrient-rich compounds. Collectively, these are achieved through processes such as milling and enrichment programs such as mixing molasses, minerals, nitrogen enrichment, etc. This chapter focuses on the potential of different crop residues as animal feed and some processing techniques that make the best use of crop residues as good unconventional feedstuffs for ruminant animals, equivalent to any conventional feed.*

**Keywords:** Alternate feed resources, Animal feed, Crop residues, Nutrients, Processing

India has a primarily agrarian economy. A significant portion of the country's land is utilized for agriculture, and many of its agro-ecological regions cultivate a broad spectrum of crops. With a production of 93.9 million tons (Mt) of wheat, 104.6 Mt of rice, 21.6 Mt of maize, 20.7 Mt of millets, 357.7 Mt of sugarcane, 8.1 Mt of fibre crops, 17.2 Mt of pulses and 30.0 Mt of oilseeds crops, in the year 2011-12, it is usual that a massive amount of crop residues are produced both on-farm and off-farm. The country produces approximately 500-550 Mt of crop residues per year in the country. Therefore, landholders are facing difficulties in managing crop residues in the country. The human population has grown four times in the last century. With a projected 9.7 billion people in the world by 2050, worldwide food consumption and the demand for meat and milk are likely to increase by as much as 73% and 58%, respectively. Improved agricultural and industrial practices have contributed to the population boom, which continues to put pressure on food supply to feed a growing population. Huge quantities of food resources will be needed, but again, the crop residues produced at these levels of global production pose major challenges.

## Availability of Crop Residues

India produces more than 500 million tons (Mt) of agricultural residue on an annual basis. The quantity of residue produced has grown significantly due to the cultivation of wheat and rice. Crop residue output varies greatly, and the use of these residue is influenced by the crops cultivated, the intensity of cropping, and the productivity across different Indian regions. About 70% of the total crop residues (352 Mt) are contributed by cereal crops (rice, wheat, maize, millets), with rice contributing 34% and wheat 22%. The excess agricultural residues—that is, the residues left over after subtracting the amount used for other purposes—are often burned on the farm. The amount of surplus crop residues available in India is estimated between 84 and 141 Mt per year where cereals crops contribute 58. As an estimate, about 70 MTs of surplus crop residue are burned annually.

## Potential of Crop Residue as Feed

Crop residues are potential source of nutrients and their beneficial effect on soil fertility and productivity could be harnessed by recycling them in to the soil. According to estimates, 30–35% of applied N & P and 70–80% of applied K accumulates in crop residues of food crops. Furthermore, crop residues are the main source of organic matter, which is essential for the sustainability of agricultural ecosystems and makes up around 40% of all dry biomass. At maturity, the vegetative components of the rice still contain around 40% of the N, 30%-35% of the P, 80-85% of the K, and 40-50% of the S that were absorbed by the rice. Likewise, 25 to 30 percent of N and P, 35 to 40 percent of S, and 75 to 75 percent of K intake is retained in wheat residue. It was found that on a dry weight basis, a ton of rice straw typically contains 5-8 kg N, 0.7-1.2 kg P, 12-17 kg K, 0.5-1 kg S, 3-4 kg Ca, 1-3 kg Mg, and 40-70 kg Si. Similarly in another study, it was estimated that one ton of wheat residue includes 4–5-kilogram N, 0.7-0.9 kg P, and 9–11 kg K. Rice straw from the North West Indian Gangetic Plain often has a greater K concentration (up to 25 kg per tone) than rice straw from other parts of India or other countries. The concentration of nutrients in crop residue is, however, influenced by soil characteristics, crop management, variety, and season. In India, the 197 Mt of rice and wheat residues produced contain around 4.1 x 106 Mt of NPK. Approximately 9-11 kg S, 100 g Zn, 777 g Fe, and 745 g Mn are also present in one ton of rice and wheat residues in addition to NPK. Thus, crop residues play a crucial role in the cycling of nutrients in addition to the role that chemical fertilizers play in crop production. Their continuous removal and burning, however, can result in nutrient net losses, which will ultimately increase the cost of nutrients in the short term and reduce soil quality and productivity in the long run.

Amongst crop varieties, the cereal crops generate large quantities of stem and leaf besides crop harvest, which become part of livestock diet for conversion into economic products. In order to provide livestock with an adequate quantity of feed during the lean season when fodder is short, these residues are utilized to their fullest potential through appropriate storage. Table 1 lists the various sources of crop residues

**Table 1:** Crop residue from different agricultural plants

| **Crop** | **By-product for feed** |
|---|---|
| Rice | Straw, bran |
| Wheat | Straw, bran |
| Barley | Straw |
| Maize plant | Stover, cobs, bran |
| Millet | Straw |
| Sorghum | Straw |
| Sugarcane | Bagasse, tops, molasses |
| Pulses | Hay, meal |
| Sunflower, olive, linseed, mustard | Cakes, straw, prunings |
| Roots and tubers | Waste |
| Vegetables and tubers | Tops, peelings |

## 1. Straw

Straw is a useful maintenance diet for ruminants in most societies across the world, however due to its poor nutritional composition to be considered as a complete ration for production animals, balancing with quality green fodder and concentrates to form total mixed ration is often recommended. The primary contributors of straw harvest, rice and wheat, with a lesser proportion originating from oat, barley, millet, and nearly other cereal crops produces high quality and palatable roughages. These straws are readily collected, handled and baled using mechanized or the conventional approach with typical haymaking equipment.

### *a. Rice straw*

Rice straw is the vegetative part of the rice plant, cut usually at grain harvest or after. Compared to other cereals, rice straw is unusual, for the fact that the stem is more digestible than leaves. It is therefore considered economic to cut it as close to the ground as possible. With traditional harvesting, the crop is often harvested when the straw is still relatively green, therefore producing better quality straw than from mature plants. Animals are more likely to eat rice straw if the time between rice harvest and straw baling is shorter than 10 days. It is recommended that bales of rice straw be prepared within 1-3 days after harvest because the ADF content increases by 5% (i.e., from 51 to 56% with 30 days), which will decrease its digestibility. But at the same time high moisture content may decrease shelf life of bales if prepared at early stage.

Rice straw contains 1–2% oxalate, 8-4% silica and 6-7% lignin. Water washing removes 30–40% of the oxalates, but at the same time, washing will also result in the loss of soluble nutrients, equal to about 10% of the original weight of straw. The effect of oxalates in the animal body can be negated if calcium and phosphorus are supplemented at 10 g and 5 g daily in animal rations, respectively. As a thumb rule, rice straw can be fed at 1.0–1.2 kg/100 kg live weight per day to ruminants. Mostly rice straw feeding is done with supplements of green fodder and concentrates.

**Table 2:** Nutrient composition of rice straw under different condition

| **Types (location and varieties)** | **Average Nutrient composition (g/kg DM)** | | | | | **Minerals (%)** | |
|---|---|---|---|---|---|---|---|
| | **OM** | **CP** | **Cellulose** | **H/cellulose** | **Lignin** | **P** | **Ca** |
| Highland | 775 | 59 | 298 | 250 | 71 | 0.14 | 0.37 |
| Low land | 779 | 52 | 288 | 261 | 70 | 0.16 | 0.28 |
| Wet season | 767 | 60 | 285 | 235 | 77 | 0.11 | 0.33 |
| Dry season | 788 | 58 | 302 | 276 | 64 | 0.14 | 0.28 |
| Mean value | 777 | 56 | 293 | 256 | 70 | 0.14 | 0.33 |

### *b. Wheat straws*

Wheat straws are important source of nutrition in traditional wheat-growing countries of Asia and Africa. Harvesting and processing technology is similar to the rice straw, but developments in harvesting methods have effects on straw quality to some extent. With the combine harvesters and grain drying, the crop is cut at a slightly mature stage, which further causes more leaf loss and straw of lower feeding value.

## 2. Stubble

Stubble comprises of the stumps of harvested crops like cereals and legumes that are left in the field after harvest. Often times, valuable feed in the form of grain and weeds are left in the stubble after the base of the crop has been harvested, especially when harvesting is done mechanically. The livestock benefits from stubble grazing because it enables them to graze selectively and likely get at least a maintenance diet from what could otherwise be a sub-maintenance feed. However, on-field grazing causes significant waste due to trampling.

## 3. Stover

Large crops like sorghum and maize have field residues that are known as "stover." In many regions of the world, these remains represent important forages. Stover is typically handled and dried in the long, unchopped state in small-scale production systems, usually by stooking in, or on, the field's boundary prior to storage. It is also ensiled and baled in large-scale processes, either with or without urea treatment. The full plant remnants (stalks, leaves, husks, and cobs) left in the field after corn is harvested are called maize stover, and it offers a lot of potential for growth and use. Many small-scale farms either graze the stover on the field after the corn harvest, while others harvest and dry in the field or at the homestead as a resource for economical winter cattle fodder. In larger farms, it is either ensiled or baled after drying. Compared to most straws, maize stover contains more nutrients.

Sweet-corn cobs, one of the corn kinds, are picked when the plant is still green and produce a substantial quantity of high-quality roughage as a by-product. After the corn has been harvested, this stover is being allowed to continue growing. Compared to stover from fully ripe crops, stover from such plants offers better feed. The study suggests that the amount of nutrients in different regions of a maize plant varies considerably. Easily digestible and better in nutrients than leaves, husks only make up around 12% of the residue left in a field. The leaves have the strength to support a mature, non-lactating cow. The nutritional composition of corn stover is given in Table 3.

Sorghum stover is also harvested as soon as the crop is harvested, ideally by cutting it while still green and it is then dried for use in corn feed in later. In some countries, grazing is practiced; however, it is not ideal due to the risk of manure and trampling-related waste.

## 4. Sugarcane byproducts

Sugarcane is harvested for production of sugar, charcoal, alcohol and conversion to bio fuel. On-farm by-products of cane harvest include cane tops, terminal leaves, nodes and bundle sheath, which forms the valuable source of animal feed. Further, cane also produces other industrial by-products such as molasses and the bagasse, but the latter has negative effect on voluntary feed intake of the overall diet due to high concentration of low fermentable fibre, thus requiring treatment for the residual sugar in the pressed stalk.

The sugarcane tops (dry matter >30%) are one of the main by-products of sugarcane milling and account for 15 to 25% of the aerial part of the plant. But they are low in protein (< 6% DM) and high in crude fibre (>30% DM). The other potential constraints attached to sugarcane top feeding are organochlorine residue and low digestibility (48–56%). In general, ruminants can be fed 1.8 to 2.5 kg DM/100 kg live weight.

Sugarcane bagasse is residual fibre resulting from the extraction of sugarcane juice. It accounts for 25–35% of processing waste and has 46% dry matter on average. Its limitations for feeding include low digestibility (30%), protein (1.8%), and fat (0.6%) on a DM basis. Further, it contains 86.9% NDS, 58.4% ADF, and 12.5% lignin. Steam processing can improve its digestibility. Sugarcane bagasse can be used at 15-20% on a total mixed ration basis for cattle.

From factory sugar production, the most important by-product is final molasses, which is produced at a rate of 3–7% of the fresh sugarcane. Molasses is the soluble residue after extraction of the sucrose from cane juice. It is a rich source of readily digestible energy as well as minerals, organic acids and other nutrients. The fermentable carbohydrates in both sugarcane juice and molasses are sucrose, glucose and fructose. It contains 70–75% dry matter, 60–70% soluble sugar, 5–6 proteins, 5% potassium, and 0.9% calcium. It can be used as

- Binding agent, anti-dust agent, and palatability enhancer: 2-5% in pellets
- Additive for silage making: poor-quality grass or a legume: 5%
- Urea carrier: combined with urea, minerals, and vitamins to make solid bricks called molasses-urea blocks or multi-nutrient blocks
- Energy source: 5–10% in the cattle concentrate mixture

Rumen microbial growth appears to be highly efficient on cane juice diets. The end-products of rumen fermentation are well balanced and therefore support high animal productivity. In monogastric such as pigs, cane juice has been used as carbohydrate source; however, its economic usage is mostly limited to the finishing stage.

## 5. Vegetable Waste/Residue

The second largest source, after cereals in human food chain, which leave behind a lot of residues, is vegetable harvest. One of the major sources of vegetable residue is the cabbage, where the discarded leaves per acre can amount to up to 6 tons of edible dry matter. An acceptable ruminant feed includes carrot tops as well as carrots that were damaged during harvest or abandoned due to low quality. With the option to be fed fresh or dry, other vegetable residues with equally significant nutritious components include those from the brassica family, such as radish tops, cauliflower, and broccoli.

In comparison to traditional green oats fodder for bucks, the nutritional value of crop residues and wastes including cauliflower leaves, cabbage leaves, pea pods, and pea vines was assessed. The concentration of cell wall components in the leaves of cauliflower and cabbage was low ($P<0.05$), whereas the concentration of CP was high ($P<0.05$), with the exception that the CP of pea pods was equivalent to that of cabbage leaves. The concentration of water-soluble carbohydrates in cabbage leaves was the highest (20.6%), while that in pea pods was the lowest (4.8%). The lowest concentration of phenolic was found in pea pods (0.3%), whereas cauliflower leaves (5.7%) and cabbage leaves (5.7%) had the highest concentrations. Except for NDF, the digestibility of nutrients in cabbage and cauliflower leaves was comparable, but it was higher ($P<0.05$) than that of other vegetable wastes and typical green oats feed. Animals fed cauliflower leaves produced the most microbial protein ($P<0.05$), followed by those fed pea pods, and bucks fed pea vines. The ME value of pea vines was much lower than that of cabbage and cauliflower leaves.

Likewise, another study was performed on mature Kurdish rams to compare potato vine to alfalfa hay as reference forage in ruminants and establish its chemical composition, mineral content, nutritional digestibility, and metabolizable energy (ME). The results showed that potato leaves had much higher DM, ash, mineral, and NDF digestibility than alfalfa hay. Potato leaves had a lower NDF, ADF organic digestibility, and ME than alfalfa hay. In light of the high nutritional content of potato leaves, they can be utilized as an alternate fodder source for ruminant nutrition.

## 6. Residues of Pulse and Legume Crops

Soybean, green and black grams, and leafy pigeon pea portions are frequently farmed pulses whose leaves and stems can be used as feed. An important byproduct of pea haulms, green vines can be utilized as silage. Useful sources of roughage include pea straw and haulms from hand-harvested soybeans. While many of these have a better feeding value than cereal straws, recovering them can be quite challenging. The leaves typically turn brown or drop off at or just before harvest in humid regions, while in drier climates they shatter. It is simpler to retrieve the leaves and stems from threshing when the crop is dried completely.

The primary residues from soybeans are the byproducts of the oil and grain harvests, such as stems, leaves, and hulls, which make up the fodder portion that can be grazed, ensiled, or dried to form hay. The leaf has a high nutritional content and exceptional digestion, and it is particularly palatable to cattle. Cows and heifers can be fed on the stubble by grazing on it or by chopping it. The leftover material from threshing soybeans, known as soybean straw, can be fed to cattle as roughage. The nutritional components of soybean straw are shown in the table 3.

## 7. Sunflower Byproducts

The primary purpose of sunflower cultivation is the generation of oil, but the residue, including the plant, the heads, and the remaining stalks, are often used as roughage for animals. Silage is typically used to feed sunflower fodder. Sunflower heads that have been threshed are a great source of animal feed, but only if they have been dried beforehand. The nutritional components of sunflower by products are shown in the table 3.

## 8. Groundnut Tops

Groundnut harvesting can result in the production of very usable hay in places with favorable drying conditions at harvest time. When the haulms start to dry out and the leaves start to turn a yellowish hue, groundnut is ready for harvest. Groundnut tops are carefully collected and dried at the homestead, on house roofs, and other sunny locations sheltered from cattle in the drier regions of Asia. They could also be piled up on stakes, allowed to dry for three to six weeks, and then threshed. The animals are fed the dried straw.

## Problems Associated with Crop Residues

Crop residues are widely used as animal feed, however there are a number of limitations which restrict their utilization. Farmers have a number of challenges when it comes to crop residue. Due to a number of factors, such as storage and transportation issues, a lack of awareness and knowledge regarding the nutritional value and potential uses of crop residues, the absence of agriculture extension services, a lack of cutting-edge technology, and a lack of farmer-level trials, the use of residues is still uncommon . Farmers lack the necessary guidance for handling and storing residues. After harvesting, they either burn the residue or plow the residue with soil.

Additionally, protein is lacking in cereal crop residue, while cell wall as neutral detergent fibre accounts up as much as 80 percent of the dry matter, which is a significant source of energy for ruminants. However, the presence of phenolic and other aromatic chemicals, commonly referred to as lignin, limits the capacity of rumen micro-organisms to digest cell wall polysaccharides (cellulose and hemicellulose). Furthermore, the sorghums are notable for poisoning with prussic acid when late rains and hot temperature promote plant stubble regrowth. Trypsin inhibitors and non-starch polysaccharides are examples of anti-nutritional factors that are produced by soybean. Feeding ruminants tubers, maize cobs, and other large food items has caused choking due to blockage of the esophagus in cases where the animals only partially succeed in swallowing solid food items like potato tubers.

Leaves of some leguminous plants might lead to cause metabolic disorders like bloat . Some plants lack certain minerals; for example, the Brassica family lacks iodine. If we don't pair them with iodine supplements, it is a goitrogenic crop. Ruminants will occasionally graze on corn cobs, turnips, tubers, and bulbs. These substantial food bits lodge in the esophagus and obstruct the digestive tract. The inclusion of anti-nutritional substances like caffeine, tannins, and phenolics may also be an issue; however most of these elements may be eliminated or at least decreased through some sort of treatment, which also rises the overall cost of the final product. Crop residues have less nutritive values and high fibre content as compared to fresh green fodders. For example, straws have only 4-5% average crude protein and 1.5-1.6 Mcal/kg ME. Fresh leaves of vegetables especially cabbage, cauliflower, potatoes, and carrot, an average of 16-17% crude protein (as % of their DM) and 1.8-1.9 Mcal/kg ME is present, which is sufficient for maintenance requirement of animals. These wastes have high moisture content, being highly fermentable and rapidly perishable, which is the most important limitation for its further utilization in animal feeding. Therefore, the quality of the crop residues as readily available animal nutrition source is a strong focus of research and development.

**Table 3:** Nutrition profile of different crop residues, % DM basis

| Nutrient value | Wheat by product | | Corn stover | | Sugarcane plant | | | | Sunflower plant | | | |
|---|---|---|---|---|---|---|---|---|---|---|---|---|
| | **Straw** | **Fresh forage** | **Dried** | **Fresh** | **Whole plant** | **Stalk** | **Leaves fresh** | **Leaves dried** | **Forage (whole plant)** | **Heads after Threshing** | **Stover (stalk and heads)** | **Silage** |
| Dry matter (% as fed) | 91.0 | 29.5 | 92.9 | 28.9 | 22.6 | 38.8 | 42.4 | 85.6 | 15.8 | 89.2 | 75.8 | 21.6 |
| Crude protein | 3.0-4.0 | 11.0 | 3.7 | 6.9 | 4.1 | 2.5 | 5.2 | 2.2 | 13.0 | 9.8 | 5.7 | 12.0 |
| Crude fibre | 41.5 | 28.0 | 42.4 | 30.1 | 34.0 | 24.0 | 33.7 | 37.8 | 25.0 | 19.9 | 48.1 | 24.6 |
| Neutral detergent fibre | 77.5 | 56.4 | 82.4 | 65.5 | 50.2 | 42.5 | 71.7 | 75.4 | 39.6 | 44.3 | 66.9 | 42.1 |
| Acid detergent fibre | 50.0 | 31.9 | 53.2 | 35.9 | 29.7 | 27.3 | 38.9 | 43.2 | 35.9 | 26.3 | 56.6 | 34.9 |
| Lignin | 7.2 | 4.6 | 8.4 | 4.8 | 4.2 | 3.8 | 5.5 | 5.7 | 9.7 | 9.9 | 15.7 | 11.2 |
| Ether extract | 1.4 | 2.7 | 0.6 | 1.2 | 1.7 | 1.5 | - | - | 2.2 | 4.2 | 1.5 | 5.0 |
| Ash | 6.7 | 8.2 | 6.6 | 6.7 | 7.0 | 4.6 | 5.1 | 7.3 | 13.1 | 10.4 | 8.4 | 12.2 |
| Gross energy (MJ/kg DM | 4.8 | 3.8 | 92.9 | 28.9 | 18.2 | 18.1 | - | - | 17.3 | 17.7 | 18.3 | 18.0 |
| Calcium, ppm | 0.7 | 2.6 | 2.9 | 3.7 | 1.9 | 1.6 | - | - | 17.5 | 14.7 | 11.2 | 14.1 |
| Phosphorus, ppm | 11.2 | | 0.7 | 2.0 | 1.1 | 1.1 | - | - | 3.1 | 3.7 | 0.8 | 2.8 |

So, feeding these residues untreated could impede animal acceptance, and subsequently animal performance. Therefore, having appropriate information on the quality and quantity of feedstuff in relation to the nutrient requirement of species/breed of animals could make these residues fulfil most dietary requirement of the animals at relatively cheaper expenses. Collectively these are achieved through processes such as milling and enrichment programs such as mixing molasses, minerals, nitrogen enrichment, etc.

## Processing Crop Residue for Better Utilization

### Crop Residue Treatment

Considering most of the aforementioned problems, many new techniques have been developed to increase the efficiency of utilization of crop residues and by-products of agriculture. There are four basic means of treatment; physical, chemical, physico-chemical and biological. These methods collectively help in improving nutrient availability to the animals through better digestibility. The physical treatment is mostly to reduce the residue size and increase surface area exposed to the digestive enzymes in animal body, while other three means are to enhance the process of digestion in the animal body.

It has been recommended that urea treatment of straw for storage and urea molasses treatment of straw for fresh feeding for better utilization in animals.

a) ***Urea treatment of straws:*** Dissolve 14 kg urea in 200 L of water and sprinkle the water on 400kg of wheat bhusa, rice straw or maize stover thoroughly and stack it for 9 days after pressing it well. After 9 days, the stacked wheat bhusa should be dried and can be fed to the animals. During this process, the temperature inside the stake increases to 50–55 °C when the lignocellulosic bond of straw is broken, resulting in enhanced digestibility of fibre or wheat straw. During the process, microbes present on wheat straw/rice straw break down the urea to ammonia and then use this ammonia for their own protein synthesis. Hence, urea treatment enhances the digestible crude protein content of wheat straw up to 3 percent and helps in saving concentrate mixtures for maintenance purposes. The method, benefits and precaution for urea treatment of straw is given in Figure 1.

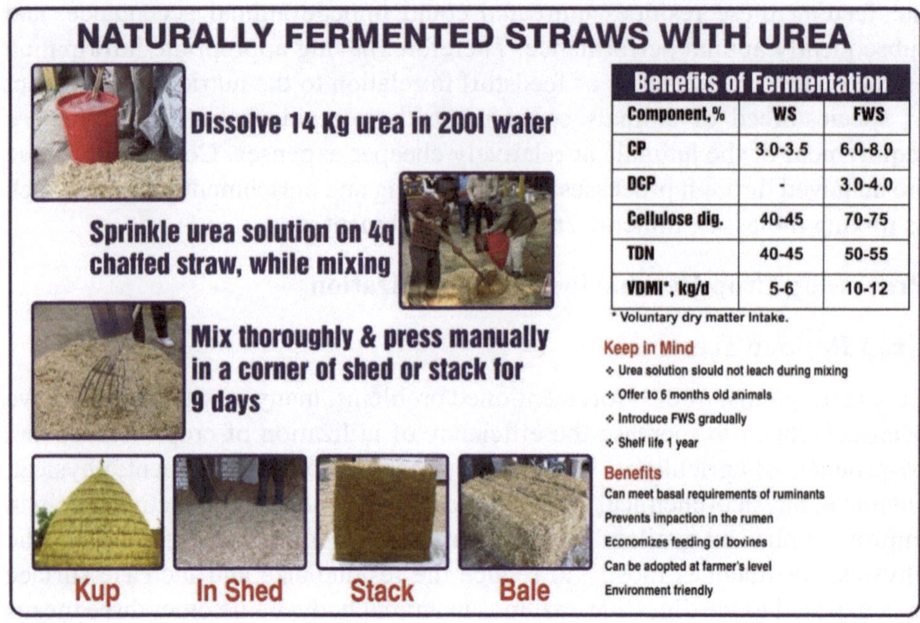


| Component,% | WS | FWS |
|---|---|---|
| CP | 3.0-3.5 | 6.0-8.0 |
| DCP | - | 3.0-4.0 |
| Cellulose dig. | 40-45 | 70-75 |
| TDN | 40-45 | 50-55 |
| VDMI*, kg/d | 5-6 | 10-12 |

**Figure 1:** Urea treatment of straws and stovers

b) ***Urea-molasses-straw feeding:*** About 1.0 kg of urea and 3.0 kg of molasses should be dissolved in 30 L of water and can be sprayed or mixed over 100 kg of chopped rice straw or wheat straw. Then mix it thoroughly and offer it to the animals in a total mixed ration. Guru Angad Dev Veterinary and Animal Sciences University, Ludhiana, utilizes urea-molasses-rice straw since 2020 for all classes of animals without any negative effect on the health, productivity, or reproductive potential of lactating animals.

## Factors Affecting Quality and Quantity of Crop Residue

The quantity of available crop residues is affected by all the factors that normally affect the yield of a crop. Animals' selective grazing habit is another factor, which leads to utilizing only certain parts or specific fractions of crop residues.

Trampling contributes to the loss of edible material during grazing. Collecting the residues and processing it (e.g., milling) increases the amount of residue ingested by the animal, but is associated with reduced animal performance because animals are forced to eat lower quality material. A number of factors affect the quality of residues, including:

a) Leaching of nutrients and damage by rain can severely reduce the nutritional value of crop residues.

b) Mode of harvesting has been shown to affect quality of residues significantly.

c) Cultivar plays a great role.

d) Plant density and crop yield, where low crop harvest produces higher quality residues because nutrients were not translocated from the stem and leaf to the grain.

Beside these factors, the technical means to improve intake as well as quality include supplementation with additives, such as spraying residues with molasses or feeding a rumen- stimulating lick such as Urea molasses brick.

## Conclusion and Recommendations

Crop residues are a valuable source of animal feed and utilizing the residues by grazing is very effective in returning plant nutrients to the soil. Sweet potato vine and broccoli by-products can replace the conventional concentrate and could be fed with poor quality hay to prevent body weight loss of an animal in the absence of other feed supplements. Efforts should be made to help the farmers to solve their feed problems mainly focus on improving methods of harvesting, handling, processing and incorporating crop residues into a year-round feed budget. Animals should be provided with supplementations while offering crop wastes and residues particularly with those nutrients/ minerals which are deficient in crops. Crop residues can be offered with highly nutritive fodder and concentrate to cope up the deficiencies. These could be used as alternatives to roughages in lean and feed shortage periods. Previous data demonstrate that animals showed good results when they fed cabbage and other vegetable leaves as fresh fodder or in the form of silage/hay. It is concluded that agriculture field crop waste and residues like cabbage leaves, cauliflower leaves, and peapods could serve as an excellent source of nutrients for ruminants and can economize the production of animals. These results introduce several applicable techniques towards making the best use of crop residues as good unconventional feedstuffs for ruminant equivalent to any conventional feed like clover hay, maize silage or fresh fodder.

The new enrichment technologies should be utilized to make these residues to be worthy of catching market across the needy societies of the world where animal production is hampered due to feed constraints. This inevitably talks of handling the problems such as storage; complete rationing exclusively with low-cost available raw materials and the means to handle anti-nutritive factors associated with crop residues.

## Suggested Readings

Akram, M.Z. and Firincioğlu, S.Y., 2019. The use of agricultural crop residues as alternatives to conventional feedstuffs for ruminants: a review. Eurasian Journal of Agricultural Research, 3(2), pp.58-66.

Aravani, V.P., Sun, H., Yang, Z., Liu, G., Wang, W., Anagnostopoulos, G., Syriopoulos, G., Charisiou, N.D., Goula, M.A., Kornaros, M. and Papadakis, V.G., 2022. Agricultural and livestock sector's residues in Greece & China: comparative qualitative and quantitative characterization for assessing their potential for biogas production. Renewable and Sustainable Energy Reviews, 154, p.111821.

Bhandari, B., 2019. Crop residue as animal feed. Paper Review, pp.1-18.

Cassida, K.A., Barton, B.A., Hough, R.L., Wiedenhoeft, M.H. and Guillard, K., 1994. Feed intake and apparent digestibility of hay-supplemented brassica diets for lambs. Journal of Animal Science, 72(6), pp. 1623-1629.

Dobermann, A. and Witt, C. 2000. The potential impact of crop intensification on carbon and nitrogen cycling in intensive rice systems. (In): Carbon and Nitrogen Dynamics in Flooded Soils. Kirk, G. J. D. and Olk, D. C. (Eds.). International Rice Research Institute, Los Banos, Philippines. pp. 1-25.

Kumar, B., Bhardwaj, N., Agrawal, K., Chaturvedi, V. and Verma, P., 2020. Current perspective on pretreatment technologies using lignocellulosic biomass: An emerging biorefinery concept. Fuel Processing Technology, 199, p.106244.

Loehr, R., 2012. Agricultural waste management: problems, processes, and approaches. Elsevier.

Lukuyu, B., Franzel, S., Ongadi, P.M. and Duncan, A.J., 2011. Livestock feed resources: Current production and management practices in central and northern rift valley provinces of Kenya. Livestock Research for Rural Development, 23(5), p.112.

Megersa, T., Urge, M. and Nurfeta, A., 2013. Effects of feeding sweet potato (Ipomoea batatas) vines as a supplement on feed intake, growth performance, digestibility and carcass characteristics of Sidama goats fed a basal diet of natural grass hay. Tropical Animal Health and Production, 45, pp.593-601.

Mottaleb, K.A., Fatah, F.A., Kruseman, G. and Erenstein, O., 2021. Projecting food demand in 2030: Can Uganda attain the zero-hunger goal? Sustainable Production and Consumption, 28, pp.1140-1163.

Pacahuri, R.K., Yadav, R.B., Nath, A., Patel, J.N., Alam, M.S. and Kumar, A., 2023. In-situ Rice Residue Management Practices and Its Impact on Climate, Soil Fertility and Crop Productivity: A Review. Int. J. Plant Soil Sci, 35(17), pp.184-195.

Salehi, S., Lashkari, S., Abbasi, R.E. and Kamangar, H. 2014. Nutrient digestibility and chemical composition of potato (Solanum tuberosum L.) vine as alternative forage in ruminant diets. Agricultural Communications, 2(1), pp.63-66.

Sharma, U.C., 2016. Crop residues in India: extent, management, uses and implications. Compendium of lecture notes of summer school. Recent approaches in crop residue management and value addition for entrepreneurship development, July, 14, pp.13-21.

Singh, Y. and Sidhu, H.S., 2014. Management of cereal crop residues for sustainable rice-wheat production system in the Indo-Gangetic plains of India. Proceedings of the Indian National Science Academy, 80(1), pp.95-114.

Wadhwa, M., Kaushal, S. and Bakshi, M.P.S., 2006. Nutritive evaluation of vegetable wastes as complete feed for goat bucks. Small Ruminant Research, 64(3), pp.279-284.

Wadhwa, M. and Bakshi, M.P.S., 2013. Utilization of fruit and vegetable wastes as livestock feed and as substrates for generation of other value-added products. Rap Publication, 4(2013), p.67.

# 4

# Artificial Intelligence in Modern Dairy Farming

***Suresh Kumar***

*Department of Livestock Production Management, College of Veterinary Science, Guru Angad Dev Veterinary and Animal Sciences University Ludhiana, Pubjab*

## Abstract

*Artificial Intelligence (AI) is a new data driven technology which needs to bring in a dairy sector for improving the livestock productivity and eventually, it will provide new hope and open prospects for the overall quality and progress of the dairy industry. This technology has a huge potential for monitoring, forecasting as well as optimizing farm animal growth, health, physical, physiological conditions of dairy animals and has multiple applications like monitoring the activity, inactivity period, rumination and disease management in dairy animals which will boost the milk production. This knowledge-based technology has a tremendous potential and could confront the existing lacunas in dairy farming and thus indirectly can strengthen the dairy industry. Artificial Intelligence is a set of electronic tools and methods for managing* livestock. *It involves automated monitoring of animals to improve their production/reproduction, health, welfare, and impact on the environment. AI technologies include* cameras, microphones, *and other* sensors *for* tracking livestock, *as well as accompanying* computer software. *The data recorded can be either quantitative or qualitative, and/or address* sustainability. *The adoption of AI is restricted to some of the farmers thereby, additional research needs to be undertaken to examine the adoption process for not only successful adoption of technology, but also to solve the issues associated with the technology adoption. Further, right extension approaches and advisory services for the farmers interested needs to be undertaken for its effective application. It will bring new era in the dairy sector to augment the livestock farmers' income, which will certainly improve the health and productivity of the livestock farmers.*

**Keywords:** Activity, Artificial Intelligence, Dairy, Software, Technology

Currently, the milk production of country is 221.06 million tonnes (2021-22) and the target is 300 million tonnes by 2023-24. The livestock sector contributed nearly 5.21% of total gross value added (GVA) and 28.36% of the agriculture and allied sectors GVA. Thus, there is a huge gap between demand and supply, therefore with the requirements of better yield from the dairy animals, we need more better and advanced options. Artificial intelligence (AI) is one of such options which can be exploited in dairy industry. Artificial Intelligence can be a game-changer for the dairy farming in India and it can emerge as a tool that empowers farmers in monitoring, forecasting as well as optimizing the farm animal growth. It can predominantly change the scenario of dairy farmers by maintaining the health, physiological and physical conditions of dairy-cows. This knowledge-based technology has a huge potential and could confront the loopholes in dairy farming and thus indirectly can strengthen the dairy industry. In dairy farming AI has multiple applications like monitoring the activities of the dairy-cows, boosting the milk production and farm productivity, detection of mastitis in dairy-cows and developing the smart cow houses powered by image analysis.

AI enables the dairy farmers to determine whether the cow is ill, ready to breed or has become less productive. The AI also sends alerts to the farmer about the change in the cow's behavior allowing human intervention where needed. Regular 24x7 monitoring of dairy animals is the key for successful dairy farming, however, traditional methods of monitoring relied on visual observation, but it was not very efficient due to the lack of time and human resources. Without AI, it would be almost impossible for the farmer to keep a watchful eye on every cow in the herd. Artificial Intelligence components of the dairy automation system process the collected data to provide insights on the heat stress, change in feeding efficiency and the estrus of the cow. Diseases like sub-clinical mastitis, one of the more common diseases in the dairy industry, cost the Indian dairy industry one billion dollars annually. Eventually, it provides new hope and open prospects for the overall quality and progress in the dairy industry through a profitable business approach in dairy farming

AI is the use of technologies to measure physiological, behavioural and production indicators of individual animals to improve management strategies and farm performance. It can also be defined as information and technology-based farm management system to identify, analyse and manage variability within farm management for optimum farm performance, profitability and sustainability. AI, with specific emphasis on technologies for individual animal monitoring, aims for an ecologically and economically sustainable production of milk with secured quality, as well as a high degree of consumer and animal protection. Precision farming is based on information technology, which enables the producer to collect information and data for better decision making. AI refers to the use of technologies that makes farmers less dependent on human labour, supports them in their (daily) management, and helps them to improve their farm profitability.

Machine learning and GPS-enabled collars in dairy farming: Dairy farmers usually relies on workers to observe hundreds of dairy animals and dairy animals are notoriously stoic, often hiding symptoms of poor health from potential predators. GPS-enabled smart collars that are fitted to each dairy cow and coupled with an app that allows farmers to remotely shift virtually fence and proactively monitor their cow's health, feed, and behaviour. The motion and temperature data of the livestock collected through the sensors are transmitted to a state-of-the-art gateway, this gateway is capable of collecting the sensor output from up to 250 neck collars transmitting simultaneously, ensuring minimal information loss in the transmission. The information received from all the collars is bifurcated and the gateway sends this information to the cloud for processing via cellular technology which is easily accessible in rural areas. The cloud is where different machine learning algorithms run to provide the health status of individual cattle through a live dashboard at the dairy farm (Smart Collar, IIT Ropar). The machine learned algorithms interpret the activity status of the cattle (chewing, ruminating, resting, moving) through the accelerometer sensor readings received and also monitor the heat cycle of the cattle based on the temperature and activity status. Inferences provided by the algorithms can be monitored live on the dashboard and based on the inferences, these algorithms also provide alerts to the farmers so that they can immediately know, for example, that the cattle need medical attention, or is going into the reproductive cycle. Heat alerts are important for timely insemination. This way, the status of each individual cattle can be monitored on the dashboard and the farmer just needs to do the needful whenever he receives an alert. This saves a lot of time and also allows efficient supervision of livestock well-being.

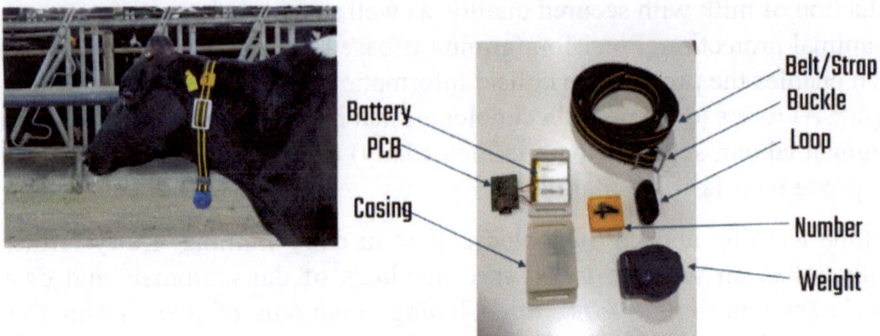


**Figure 1:** End node components for dairy animals

In practice, these advanced technologies can be used to determine optimal solutions to many animal farming problems. A few examples include finding optimal solutions to minimize costs, maximize production, increase efficiencies and create optimal diet formulations . Advanced models may even consider variables such as genetics, environment and management priorities in order to come up with relevant and contextually optimal solutions. In general, the more diverse datasets a system collects and analyses, the better are its chances of arriving at accurate and optimal solutions. Such a solution will also have the advantage of providing farmers an evidence-based or data driven solution.

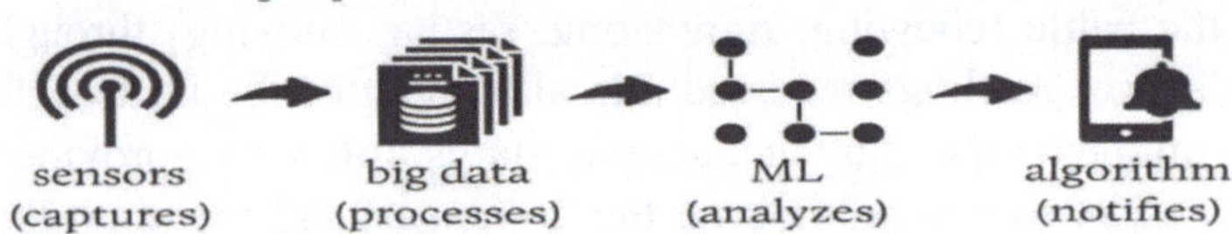


**Figure 2:** The collection of data from sensors to algorithm

**How to work with automated cattle health monitoring systems:** Data of the dairy animals through end nodes transmitted through gateway to the cloud for processing and interpretation of the data will be on the dashboard at the dairy farm.

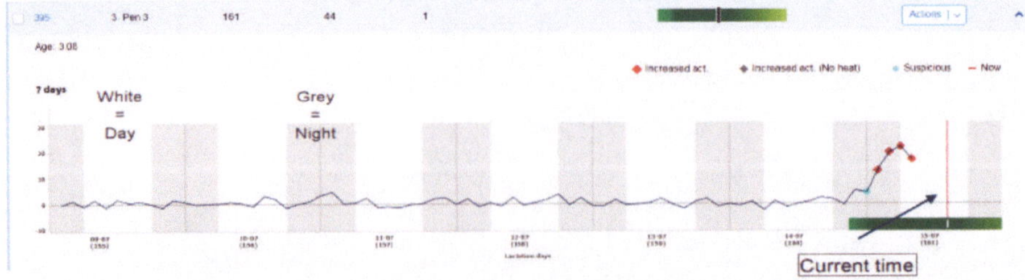

- Individual animal observation

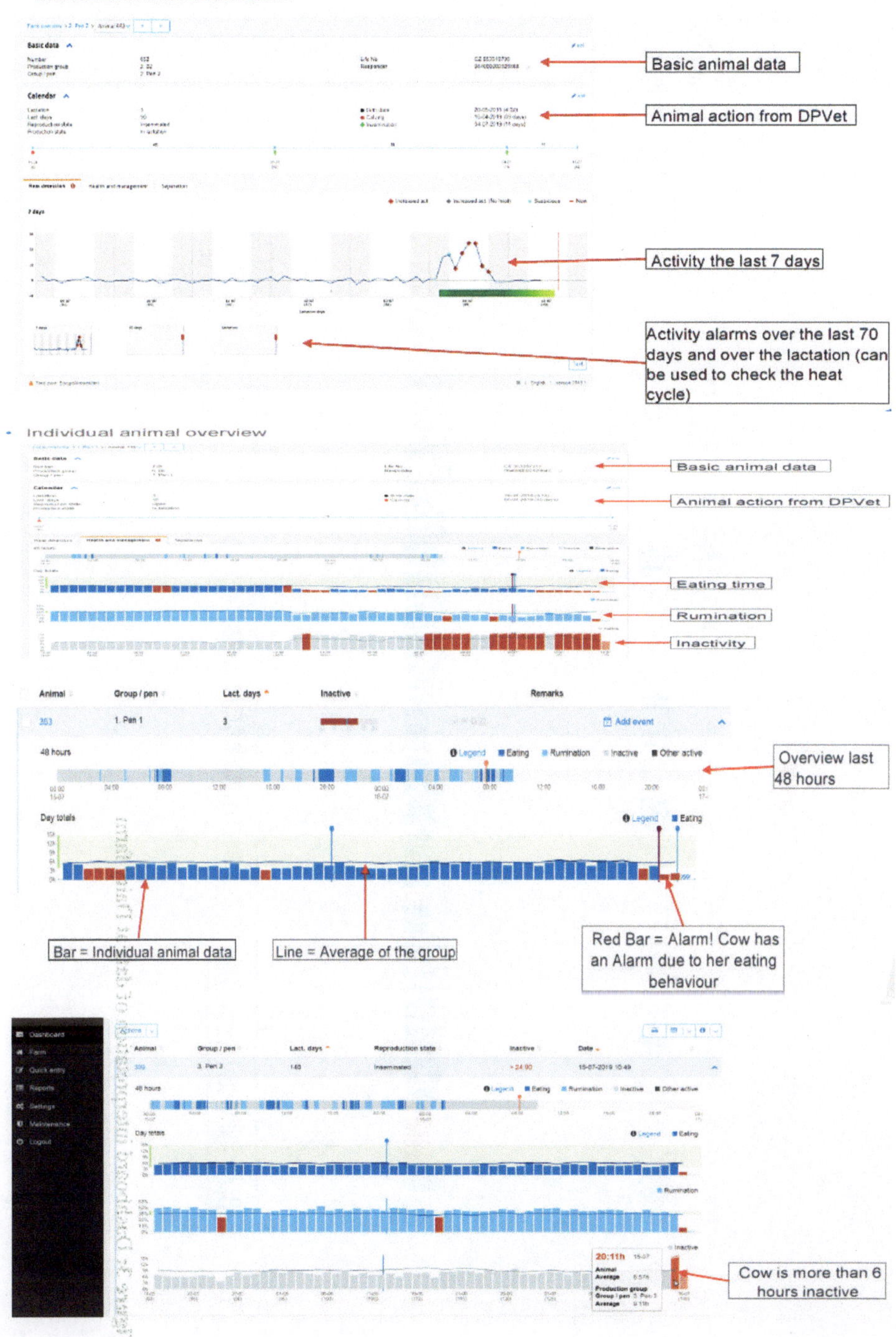

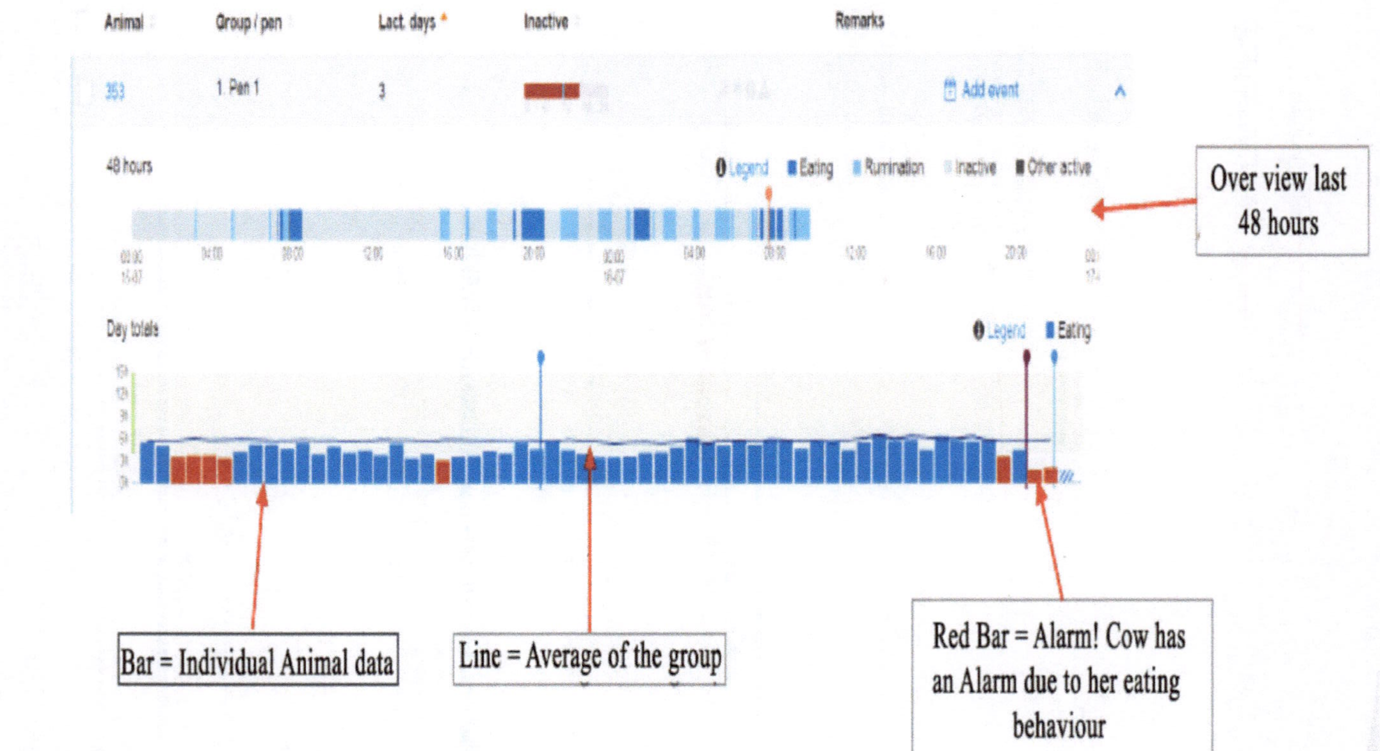


**Figure 3:** Dashboard interpretation of data at Dairy farm

Emotional communication can be a useful tool to regulate social interactions such as mating competition, play, maternal nursing, and group defence. Harmonizing the emotional behaviours of individual animals can help other farm-animals develop more empathy and other desirable traits. This may result in the entire herd developing strong social bonds and improved group coordination.

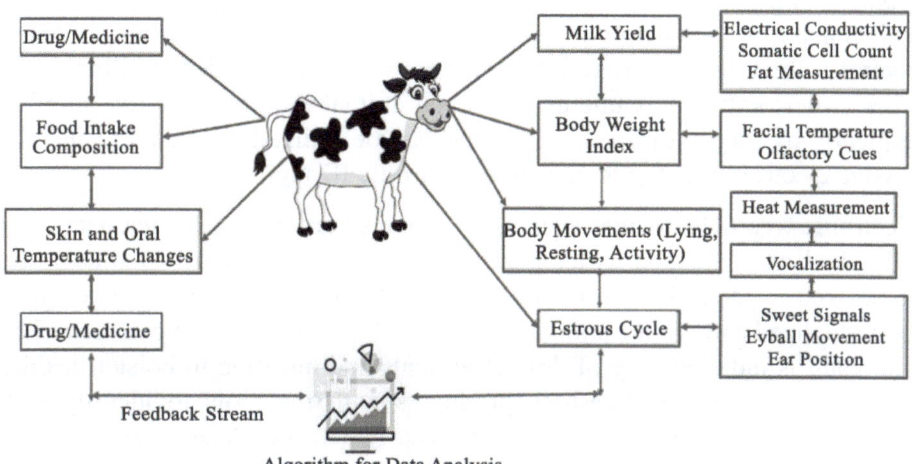


**Figure 4:** A representation of how machine learning algorithms might interpret data to create optimal growth conditions in dairy farming

Machine learned-based AI can help us identify the variables of emotional contagion based on vocalizations, olfactory cues, etc. to detect the outburst of a specific disease or stress (Figure 4). The animal farming industry is quickly becoming a hotspot for new technologies such as deep learning, AI, and ML. These smart farming technologies are being used to monitor animals , predict diseases , optimize food intake, and improve animal health .

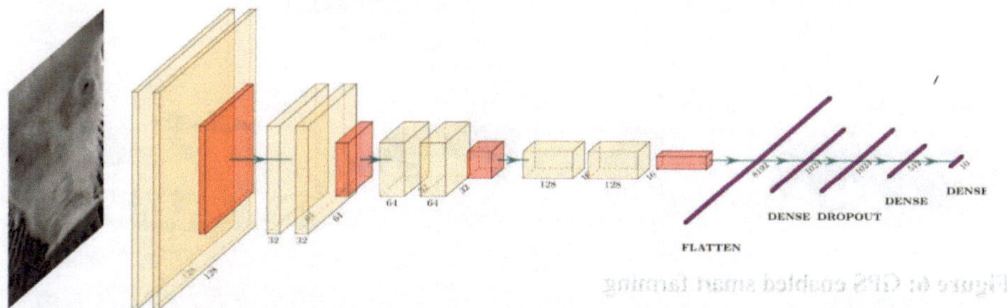


**Figure 5:** Flow diagram showing the neural network for emotional contagion of farm animals

## Economic livestock farming

Due to academic studies, the requirements of an animal are well known for each phase of its life and individual physical demands. These requirements allow the precise preparation of an optimal feed to support the animal. The requirements are oriented on the required nutrition – providing more nutrition than required make no economic sense, but providing less nutrients can be negative to the health of the animal. Precision livestock farming (PLF) starts with consistently collecting information about each animal. For this, there are several technologies: unique ID, electronic wearables to identify illness and other issues, software, cameras, etc. Each animal requires a unique number (typically by means of an ear tag). This can be utilized through a visual ID, passive electronic ID tag or an active electronic ID tag.

Electronic wearable devices such as an active smart ear tag can get data from individual animals such as temperature and activity patterns. This data can be utilized in identification of illness, heat stress, oestrous etc. This enables individualized care for the animals and methods to lower stress upon them. The end result is judicious use of drug treatments and nutrition to bolster healthy growth. This provides livestock producers with the tools to identify sick animals sooner and more accurately. This early detection leads to reduction in costs by lowering re-treatment rate and death loss, and getting animals back to peak performance faster. Data recorded by the farmer or collected by sensors is then gathered by software. Although there has been software used that was run on a single computer, it has become more common for the software to connect to the internet, so that much of the data processing can happen on a remote server. Having the software connected to the internet can also make it easier to look up information about a particular animal.

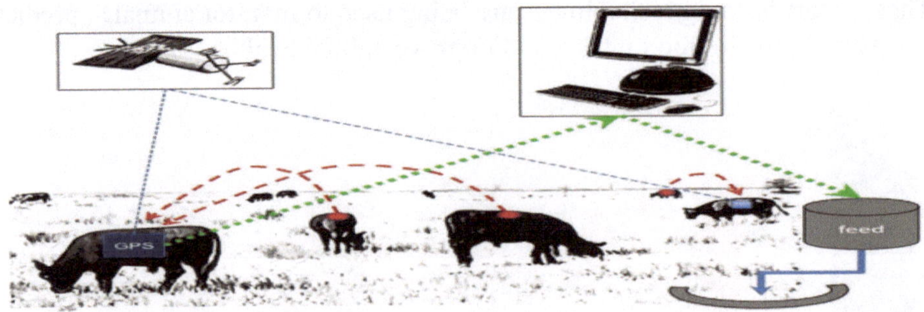


**Figure 6:** GPS enabled smart farming

## Applications of Artificial Intelligence (AI) in Livestock Farming

***Robotic Milker:*** In automatic milking, a robotic milker can be used for precision management of dairy cattle. The main advantages are time savings, greater production, a record of valuable information, and diversion of abnormal milk. Brands of robotic milkers include Lely and DeLavel.

***Milk yield and milk electrical conductivity:*** It has been observed that significant changes in milk yield and electrical conductivity can be observed as early as 10 days before diagnosis of an adverse health event. Though, PDF technologies may alert the dairy farmer at an earlier stage giving time advantage, they do not indicate what type of disease is onset. This approach also fails to detect small changes in milk yield or milk electrical conductivity that are often associated with the onset of a health disorder. Further, it has been reported that electrical conductivity along with other information (e.g., milk yield, milk flow, number of incomplete milking) may increase accuracy of detection and ability to determine early onset of mastitis.

***Automatic Feeders**:* An automatic feeder is a tool used to provide feed to cattle. It is composed of a robot (either on a rail system or self-propelled) that will feed the cattle at designated times. The robot mixes the feed ration and will deliver a programmed amount.

***Activity Collars**:* Activity collars gather biometric data from animals. Some wearable devices help farmers with estrous detection, as well as other adverse health events or conditions. The use of GPS 'collar' for livestock including dairy animals has become widespread in the last two decades. This has opened the possibility of recording detailed position information for long periods of time, thus allowing a more complete understanding of the habits and causes of spatial distribution of ruminants. Further, given the history of prices in electronic technology, it is very likely that with the proper investment in research and development, we can have cost effective herd information systems with which we will be able to see where and how all of our animals are and what they are doing at any time.

***Inline Milk Sensors**:* Inline milk sensors help farmers identify variation of components in the milk. Some sensors are relatively simple technologies that measure properties such as electrical conductivity, and others use automated sampling and reagents to provide a different measure to inform management decisions.

***Rumen pH:*** Measurement of ruminal fluid pH is a reliable and accurate diagnostic test for ruminal acidosis. Individual dairy cows exhibit tremendous variation in the degree of acidosis they experience, even when fed and managed similarly. However, rumen pH could be used as an instrument steering rumen fermentation for optimal production and health of cows. Continuous monitoring of ruminal pH is possible through wireless telemetry which has the capacity to accurately detect subacute ruminal acidosis.

***Rumination:*** The percentage of cows ruminating at any given time has been considered by many people as an indicator of herd rumen health, as ruminal pH is affected by the amount of time the cow spends ruminating. Technologies for the automatic capture of rumination would allow for easy detection of changes in both individual cow and herd rumen health, and thus allow for the diagnosis of acute acidosis. An example of this is an electronic rumination monitoring system, which would allow for easy detection of changes in both the individual cow, as well as herd rumen health, and thus, allow for the detection of a bout of acidosis.

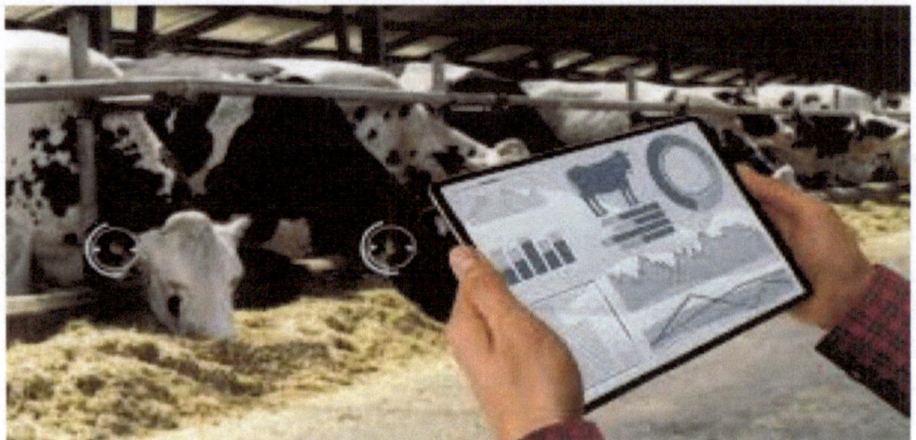

**Figure 7:** Monitoring of dairy animals through Artificial Intelligence

***Rumen temperature:*** The use of ruminal temperature in field situations depends on future development of a practical and cost effective intra-ruminal wireless telemetry temperature sensing device. They act as rumen sensors to measure temperature, pressure/motility and pH in rumen.

***Body condition score (BCS):*** Only a few dairy farmers have integrated BCS based on visual evaluation in their daily management strategy mainly because it is fairly time consuming and subjective. It has been observed that there is a strong relationship between the angles measured by video imaging and the BCS as determined by trained evaluators. Further, investigation found that measuring Backfat Thickness (BFT) by ultrasound is of added value compared with other body condition scoring systems because it is objective and precise.

Ongoing research on automation of body condition scoring suggests that it must be incorporated into decision support systems in the near future to aid producers in making operational and tactical decisions.

***EID/RFID/Electronic Identification/Electronic Ear Tages:*** Radio Frequency Identification (commonly known as RFID or EID) is applied in cattle, pigs, sheep, goats, deer and other types of livestock for individual identification. There is currently a growing trend of RFID or EID becoming mandatory for certain species. For example, Australia has made EID compulsory for cattle, as has New Zealand for deer, and the EU for sheep and goats. EID makes identification of individual animals much less error-prone. RFID enhances traceability, but it also provides other benefits such as reproduction tracking (pedigree, progeny, and productivity), automatic weighing, and drafting.

***Smart Ear Tags:*** Cattle hide their symptoms of illness from humans due to their predatory response. Smart cattle ear tags constantly gather behavioural and biometric data from cattle, allowing managers to see the exact animals that need more attention regarding their health. Smart ear tagging has been shown to be effective in identifying illness earlier and more accurately than traditional visual monitoring.

***Automated Weight Detection Cameras:*** Automated weight detection cameras can be used to calculate the pig's weight without a scale. These cameras can have an accuracy of less than 1.5 kilograms.

***Microphones to Detect Respiratory Problems:*** In the swine industry, the presence of respiratory problems must be closely monitored. There are multiple pathogens that can cause infection; however, enzootic pneumonia is one of the most common respiratory diseases in pigs caused by Mycoplasma hyopneumoniae and other bacteria. This is an airborne disease that can be easily spread due to the proximity of the pigs in the herd. Early detection is important in using fewer antibiotics and minimizing economic loss due to appetite loss of pigs. A common symptom of this is chronic coughing. A microphone can be used to detect the sound of coughing in the herd and raise an alert to the farmer.

***Climate Control:*** Thermal stress is connected to reduced performance, illness, and mortality. Depending on geographical location, and the types of animals will require different heating or ventilation systems. Broilers, laying hens, and piglets like to be kept warm. Sensors can be used to constantly receive data about the climate control in the livestock houses and the automatic feeding systems. The behaviour of animals can also be monitored.

***Poultry Industry***: In the poultry industry, unfavorable climate conditions increase the chances of behavioural, respiratory, and digestive disorders in the birds. Thermometers should be used to ensure proper temperatures, and animals should be closely monitored for signs of unsatisfactory climate.

***Infra-Red Thermography (IRT):*** Infrared thermography (IRT) absorbs infrared radiation and generates images based on the amount of heat generated. Infrared energy can be measured using an infrared camera and a specially developed analyzing software program. A major advantage of the method is that it does not require direct physical contact with the surface monitored, thus allowing remote reading of temperature distribution.

1. As a diagnostic tool. In these cases, IRT becomes a physiological imaging method. The difference of 1 °C between two anatomically symmetric regions indicates their inflammation
2. To enhance the possibilities of physical examination. In these cases, thermography can determine suspicious areas where the heat is increased or decreased.
3. In wellness programmes. In this case, animals are monitored on a routine basis once a week. Thermography can be used to detect subclinical problems, as clinical changes occur two weeks after thermographic changes

***Total Mixed Ration (TMR):*** Total Mixed Ration (TMR) can be described as a mixture of both the roughage and the processed ingredients, formulated and mixed to supply the cows' requirements, in a form that precludes selection. The TMR technology offers many advantages that lead to increased milk production.

1. Improved rumen fermentation. Cows have continuous access to a complete and balanced ration throughout the day. Thus, they tend to consume smaller but more meals per day, spread out evenly during their day. This prevents slug feeding that overloads the rumen with nutrients and unbalances the process. In contrast, rumen processes are optimized, digestibility improves, pH stabilizes and digestive upsets are minimized. This is because with each meal, the rumen microflora receives a balanced mix of all nutrients required for fermentation towards a desirable outcome.
2. Increased dry matter intake. As digestive functionality and health are sustained at high levels and in conjunction with continuous feed availability, cows consume more dry matter. Not only that, but they

cannot pick out undesirable (unpalatable, dusty, etc.) ingredients, leading to much better efficiency of feed utilization and less residual feed. In addition, as the dry matter intake is easily monitored, nutrition can be easily adjusted to match genetic potential and actual performance, not to mention the ability to perform quick nutrition challenge on-farm trials.

3. Enhanced milk production. As it can be anticipated, a healthy cow with a functioning rumen, free of digestive disorders, and exhibiting maximal feed intake will produce more milk..

## Conclusion

Although Artificial Intelligence and Machine learning algorithms have developed so fast, there is a lack of standardization in the collection and sharing of data globally. However, as more farms get connected to technology, AI and sensing technologies will start playing a more decisive role in helping farmers see patterns and solutions to pressing problems in the modern livestock farming. Artificial Intelligence may improve the productive and reproductive parameters like milk yield, better conception rate, improvement in heat detection rate, lowers the incidence of disease. Eventually, it provides new hope and open prospects for the overall quality and progress in the dairy industry through a profitable business approach in dairy farming. Artificial Intelligence in India is still restricted to some of the farmers but there are tremendous opportunities for improvements in individual animal and herd management on dairy farms. Further research and extension activities needs to be promoted in the field of Artificial Intelligence in livestock farming to augment farmers income.

## Suggested Readings

Beauchemin K and Penner G. 2009. New Developments in Understanding Ruminal Acidosis in Dairy Cows. Tri-State Dairy Nutrition Conference. April 21 and 22, 2009. pp. 1–12

Bewley J. 2009. Precision Dairy Farming: Opportunities, Challenges, and Solutions. The Dairy Practices Council, 40th Annual Conference held at Latham, NY during 4–6th November, 2009

Bewley J. 2010. Precision Dairy Farming: Advanced Analysis Solutions for Future Profitability. In: First North American Conference on Precision Dairy Management, Toranto, Canada during 2–5 March, 2010

Bewley J and Schutz M M. 2009. Potential of Using New Technology for Estimating Body Condition Scores. Eighteenth Annual Tri-State Dairy Nutrition Conference, Fort Wayne, Indiana, USA. pp. 24–37

Fredrickson B L, Branigan C, Laar H. 2005. Positive emotions broaden the scope of attention and thought-action repertoires, Cognit. Emot. 19 (3): 313–332.

Fu Q, Shen W, Wei X, Zhang Y, Xin H, Su Z and Zhao C. 2020. Prediction of the diet energy digestion using kernel extreme learning machine: a case study with Holstein dry cows, Comput. Electron. Agric. 169: 105231

Kamphuis C, Steeneveld W and Hogeveen H. 2015. Economic modelling to evaluate the benefits of precision livestock farming technologies. Pages 87–94 in Precision Farming Applications. I. Halachmi (ed.). Wageningen Academic Publishers, Wageningen, the Netherlands. EAAP/EU-PLF joint Conference, Copenhagen, Denmark

Laca E A. 2009. Precision livestock production: tools and concepts. Revista Brasileira de Zootecnia 38: 123–32

Lukas J M, Reneau J K, Wallace R, Hawkins D and Munoz-Zanzi C. 2009. A novel method of analyzing daily milk production and electrical conductivity to predict disease onset. Journal of Dairy Science 92: 5964–76

Neethirajan S. 2020. The role of sensors, big data and machine learning in modern animal farming. Sensing and Biosensing Research 29: 100367

Nikoloski S, Murphy P, Kocev D, Džeroski S and Wall D P. 2019. Using machine learning to estimate herbage production and nutrient uptake on Irish dairy farms, J. Dairy Sci. 102 (11): 10639–10656

Phillips N, Mottram T, Poppi D, Mayer D and McGowan M R. 2010. Continuous monitoring of ruminal pH using wireless telemetry. Animal Production Science 50: 72–77

Roche J R, Friggens N C, Kay J K, Fisher M W, Stafford K J and Berry D P. 2009. Invited review: Body condition score and its association with dairy cow productivity, health, and welfare. Journal of Dairy Science 92: 5769–5801

Schirmann K, von Keyserlingk M A G, Weary D M, Veira D M and Heuwieser W. 2009. Validation of a system for monitoring rumination in dairy cows. Journal of Dairy Science 92: 6052– 55.

Spilke J and Fahr R. 2003. Decision support under the conditions of automatic milking systems using mixed linear models as part of a precision dairy farming concept. Pages 780–785 in EFITA 2003 Conference, Debrecen, Hungary

Špinka M. 2012. Social dimension of emotions and its implication for animal welfare. Appl. Anim. Behav. Sci. 138 (3–4) 170–181

VanderWaal K, Morrison R B, Neuhauser C, Vilalta C, Perez A M. 2017. Translating big data into smart data for veterinary epidemiology. Front. Vet. Sci. 4: 110

Weary D M, Huzzey J M and von Keyserlingk M A G. 2009. Using behaviour to predict and identify ill health in animals. Journal of Animal Science, 87: 770–77

Wolfert S, Ge L, Verdouw C, Bogaardt M J. 2017. Big data in smart farming–a review, Agric. Syst. 153 69–80

# 5

# Advancements in Pregnancy Detection in Farm Animals

***Ashok K. Balhara, Suman Sangwan and Sajjan Singh***

*Animal Physiology and Reproduction Division, ICAR-Central Institute for Research on Buffaloes, Hisar, Haryana*

## Abstract

*Field-ready pregnancy diagnostic tests are an important tool for improving reproductive performance in livestock. They help optimize breeding programs, resource allocation, and decision-making processes, leading to better economic outcomes and sustainable livestock production systems. Pregnancy diagnosis is an important tool for improving reproductive performance in livestock for several reasons: timely management, optimized breeding programs, resource allocation, lower costs, genetic improvement, labour efficiency, stress reduction, health management, data-driven decision making, and economic impact. Early pregnancy diagnosis is often considered important information for shortening the calving period, but none of the current methods are suitable as an ideal test for early pregnancy diagnosis due to limited accuracy, applicability only at later stages, and the need for costly equipment and laboratory facilities. Advances in molecular techniques and their application in animal research have raised new hopes for the search for biomarkers of pregnancy in animals. Urinary metabolites can be used to assess healthy pregnancies in animals, and sensor-based equipment is being miniaturized for field use.*

**Keywords:** Pregnancy diagnosis, Urinary metabolite, Precision farming

Field-ready pregnancy diagnostic tests are an important tool for improving reproductive performance in livestock. They help optimize breeding programs, resource allocation, and decision-making processes, leading to better economic outcomes and sustainable livestock production systems. Pregnancy diagnosis is an important tool for improving reproductive performance in livestock for several reasons:

1) ***Timely management**:* early and accurate pregnancy diagnosis allows farmers and livestock producers to make timely decisions about the management of pregnant and non-pregnant animals. This includes adjusting feeding regimes, providing appropriate veterinary care, and establishing breeding plans.

2) ***Optimized breeding programs:*** In livestock, controlling the timing of pregnancies is critical to maintaining a well-organized breeding program. With accurate pregnancy testing, farmers can identify non-pregnant animals and breed them back earlier, optimizing resource utilization and shortening the generation interval.

3) ***Resource allocation:*** early identification of non-pregnant animals helps avoid unnecessary allocation of resources such as feed and health care to animals that will not produce offspring in the current cycle. This efficient allocation of resources is essential to maintaining a cost-effective production system.

4) ***Lower costs:*** unproductive animals consume resources without contributing to farm productivity. By quickly identifying non-pregnant animals, farmers can avoid the cost of keeping these animals during their non-productive period.

5) ***Genetic improvement:*** for livestock programs focused on genetic improvement, accurate pregnancy diagnosis is critical. It enables the selection and promotion of animals with desirable traits for breeding purposes, thus accelerating genetic progress.

6) ***Labour efficiency:*** traditional methods of pregnancy diagnosis, such as manual rectal palpation or ultrasound, are labour intensive and require skilled personnel. On-site usable pregnancy tests simplify the process and allow non-professionals to perform the tests accurately, saving time and labour costs.

7) ***Stress reduction*****:** handling and transporting animals for pregnancy diagnosis can be stressful, especially for pregnant animals. Field testing can be done in the field, which minimizes stress to the animals and can reduce the risk of pregnancy loss due to stressors.

8) ***Health management*****:** pregnant animals often have different health requirements than non-pregnant animals. Accurate pregnancy diagnosis helps ensure that pregnant animals receive appropriate health and nutritional care, which in turn contributes to the overall health and well-being of the herd.

9) ***Data-driven decision making***: accurate pregnancy diagnosis provides farmers with reliable data from which to make informed decisions about culling, replacement and future breeding plans. This data-driven approach increases the overall efficiency and sustainability of the livestock operation.

10) ***Economic Impact***: Reproductive performance directly impacts the economic viability of livestock operations. Maximizing the number of productive pregnancies while minimizing the number of unproductive cycles can significantly impact farm profitability.

Early pregnancy diagnosis is often considered important information for shortening the calving period-identifying open animals, timely treatment, and restocking to maintain an optimal postpartum calving period. However, none of the current methods are suitable as an ideal test for early pregnancy diagnosis because of limited accuracy, applicability only at later stages, and the need for costly equipment and laboratory facilities. For this reason, research to develop novel early pregnancy detection methods for livestock has always been followed with great interest in the animal sciences. Advances in molecular techniques and their application in animal research have raised new hopes for the search for biomarkers of pregnancy in animals.

The early embryonic period in cattle is described as approximately 42 days after insemination (Committee on Reproductive Nomenclature, 1972) and includes a series of events beginning with fertilization and culminating in implantation (Table 1). After implantation, embryonic losses due to non-infectious causes are rare, and pregnancy becomes increasingly certain. Many methods of pregnancy diagnosis, both direct and indirect, are used in cattle; none of them can yet be considered the ideal method of pregnancy diagnosis because of its limitations. Advances in molecular techniques such as proteomics and their application in animal research have opened up the possibility for researchers to search for biomarkers of pregnancy in these animals.

**Table 1:** Important events during early embryonic period

| Day of Pregnancy | Event |
|---|---|
| Day 0-1 | Fertilization, single-cell embryo (zygote) in oviduct |
| Day 2 | Early cleavages in the oviduct (upto 8 cell stage), activation of embryonic genome |
| Day 3-4 | Embryo enters the uterus |
| Day 5-6 | 16-32 cell zona-enclosed embryo progressing into compact morula stage |
| Day 7-8 | Formation of a blastocoele with differentiation of embryonic cells |

| Day of Pregnancy | Event |
|---|---|
| Day 9-10 | Blastocyst expansion and hatching from the zona pellucida |
| Day 11-15 | Blastocyst elongation from tubular to a filamentous structure |
| Day 14-19 | Maternal recognition of pregnancy |
| Day 19-20 | Implantation begins |
| Day 21 | Caruncles–cotyledons appear |
| Day 22-41 | Implantation progresses |
| Day 42 | Implantation completed |

## Tools in Pregnancy Biomarker Discovery

The current "omics" era has given a major boost to the field of proteomics and metabolomics, with significant advances in analytical platforms such as chromatographic or electrophoretic separation with integrated mass spectrometry (MS), fluorescence-based methods, and nuclear magnetic resonance (NMR) spectroscopy combined with state-of-the-art bioinformatics tools to achieve high sensitivity with appropriate precision. Metabolomics is an emerging branch of "omics," defined as the global analysis of small molecules (metabolites) that involves identification, characterization, and quantification in a biological sample such as a cell, tissue, biofluid, or organ. A method for pregnancy diagnosis must be based on one or more changes in maternal physiology related to the developmental profile of the embryo. Accordingly, measurement of peripheral concentrations of progesterone, pregnancy-associated glycoproteins (PAGs), and early pregnancy factor are among the methods commonly used to detect pregnancy in cattle, each with its own advantages and limitations. In addition, in recent years, the opportunity to use maternal/foetal metabolic traits to define new biomarkers and develop new methods for non-invasive pregnancy monitoring aimed at early pregnancy detection and prediction has been recognised.

The main analytical platforms for metabolomics are nuclear magnetic resonance spectroscopy (NMR) and mass spectrometry (MS). Of these, several MS modalities, including liquid chromatography- MS (LC - MS) and gas chromatography- MS (GC- MS), are the mainstays of current metabolomics analyses. The high applicability of LC - MS - NMR permeates the field of metabolomics due to its high spectral resolution and great metabolite identification capabilities.

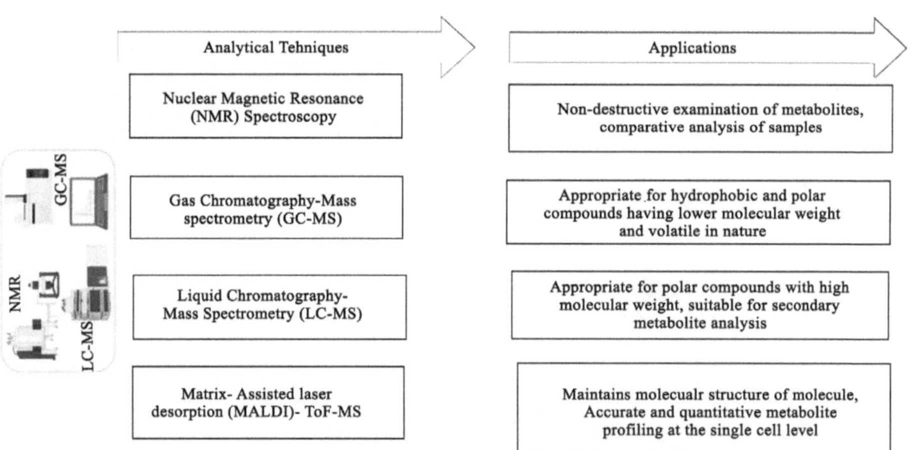


**Figure 1:** Analytical techniques and their applications in biomarker discovery

## Research on Pregnancy Diagnosis at ICAR-CIRB Hisar

At ICAR-CIRB, laboratory studies were initiated in buffalo urine, initially using proteomics and later metabolomics platforms to decipher information on differential expression of metabolites depending on pregnancy status. Experiments were performed in which buffaloes were artificially inseminated and urine was collected in sterile collection containers. These urine samples were processed in the manner indicated:

***Protein extraction*** – Total protein in urine was precipitated with ammonium sulphate/ trichloroacetic acid/ acetone. Alternatively, samples were concentrated by freeze drying followed by precipitation of proteins and peptides. These protein precipitates were analysed by 2DE - mass spectrometry-based proteomics.

***Extraction of metabolites*** - Volatile, hydrophilic and hydrophobic compounds from buffalo urine samples were collected in appropriate polar and non-polar solvents. The samples thus prepared were analysed by deuterium (1H) NMR technique to study the differences in composition depending on the gestation status of the animals. Metabolite profiling and subsequent bioinformatics were performed using the Chenomx and MestReNovo 6.0.2-5475 software programmes, and the Human Metabolome Database (HMDB) and Kyoto Encyclopaedia of Genes and Genomes (KEGG) online databases were used to identify metabolites.

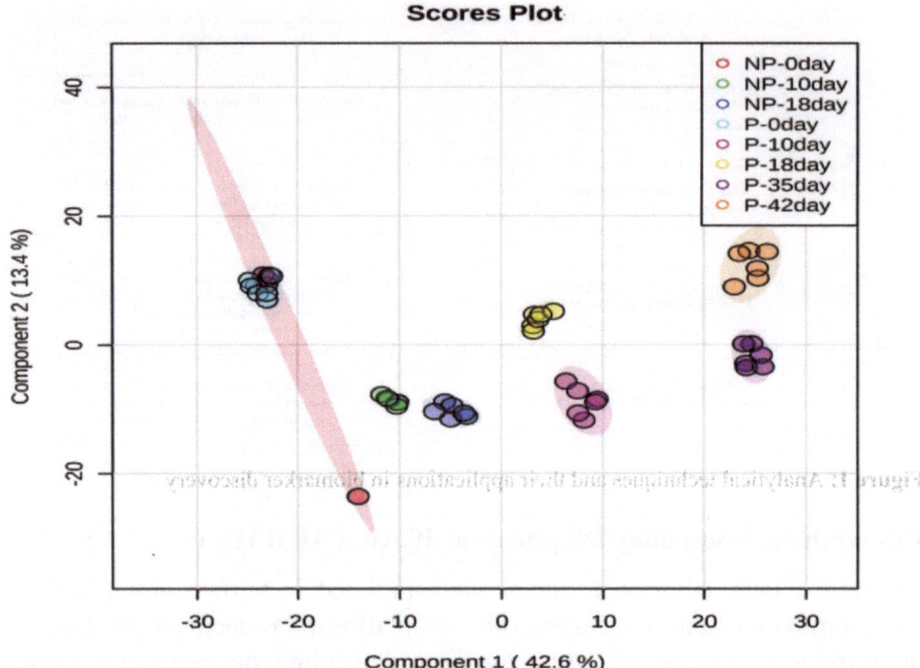


**Figure 2:** D score plot of PLS-DA analysis of different groups in different days of early pregnancy

The selected identified metabolites were later validated by gas chromatography-mass spectrometry GC-MS, LC-MS, HPLC, infrared spectroscopy (IR Spectroscopy), thin layer chromatography (TLC) and colour tests. NMR studies of urine revealed that there are numerous metabolites that are present in good usable quality and have medical, agricultural, and industrial applications.

- ***Chemical Testing*:** The magic of chemistry can be observed in the test tube by applying some chemical reactions that give a certain colour to certain functional groups in the animal fluid. The results, interpreted based on the above methods, specify some functional groups that are present in pregnant animals and absent in non-pregnant animals. The application of reagents to urine samples of animals and the specific colour difference in the test tube can be an indication of the reproductive status of the animal. The colour also has some precipitates that open a new way of improvement, such as a strip-based or sensor-based method that is farmer-friendly and easy to use.

## Novel Methods for Identification of Pregnancy/Open Animals

### 1. In Line-milk Progesterone Sensors

Progesterone is indeed a commonly used hormone to assess reproductive status in mammals including humans. In cattle, progesterone is produced by the corpus luteum, a transient endocrine structure formed in the ovary after ovulation. In pregnant cows, the corpus luteum continues to produce progesterone to maintain pregnancy. However, in non-pregnant cows, progesterone levels decrease as the corpus luteum recedes.

Progesterone tests are usually performed about 18 to 24 days after insemination or mating. If the progesterone level is low, it indicates that the cow is not pregnant and the corpus luteum has regressed. This information helps in the early detection of non-pregnant cows and allows for timely rebreeding if needed. The inline milk sensors are integrated into the milking process and allow continuous and non-invasive monitoring of progesterone levels in milk. They provide real-time or near real-time information on the reproductive status of cows and enable farmers to make informed breeding management decisions. Milk progesterone sensors are specialized devices that measure the concentration of progesterone, an important reproductive hormone, in the milk of farm animals. Progesterone plays a crucial role in the oestrus cycle and pregnancy of female animals.

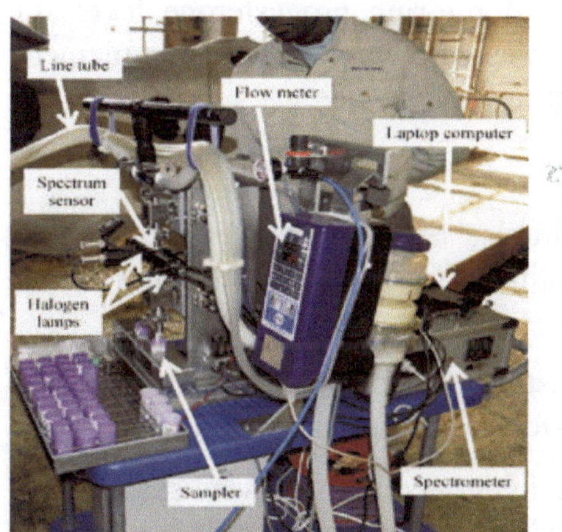


Cow Milk Progesterone Concentration Assessment during Milking Using Near-infrared Spectroscopy

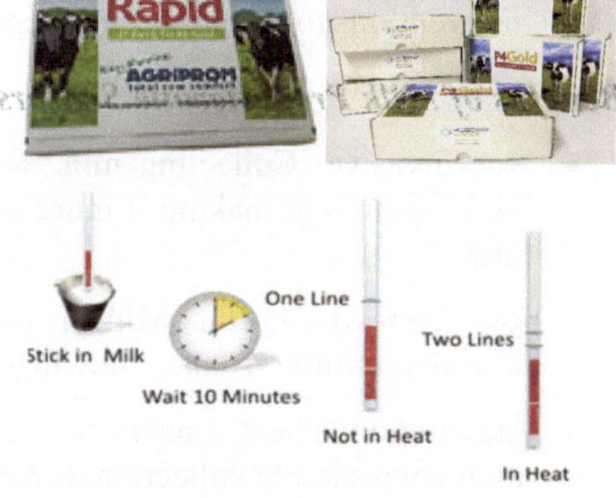


Dipstick test for progesterone

**Figure 3:** Working Principle of Milk Progesterone Sensors

Milk progesterone sensors are based on the principle of immunoassays, in which there is an interaction between progesterone molecules and specific antibodies. Antibodies are proteins that can bind to progesterone with high specificity. These sensors are designed to detect the progesterone-antibody interaction and convert it into a measurable signal, often by optical or electrochemical methods.

A. ***Assessment of reproductive status:*** Progesterone concentration in the milk sample is quantified by the sensor. Progesterone concentration in milk varies during the oestrus cycle and pregnancy. The following describes how milk progesterone sensors can be used to assess reproductive status:

B. ***Monitoring the estrous cycle:*** progesterone levels increase after ovulation and remain elevated during the luteal phase of the estrous cycle. Monitoring progesterone levels helps determine when the cow is in the luteal phase, indicating that she is not in estrus (in heat) and not ready to breed. This information is important to optimize the timing of artificial insemination.

C. ***Detection of Pregnancy:*** When a cow becomes pregnant, progesterone levels remain elevated throughout pregnancy. Detection of consistently high levels of progesterone in milk can serve as an indicator of pregnancy.

D. ***Identifying Anoestrous Animals:*** Monitoring progesterone levels in milk can help identify anoestrous cows, allowing farmers to implement interventions to restore normal reproductive cycles.

### *Benefits of Milk Progesterone Sensors*

- Non-Invasive: Collecting milk samples is less invasive compared to blood sampling, making it more suitable for routine monitoring on the farm.
- Real-Time Monitoring: Milk progesterone sensors can provide real-time or near-real-time results, allowing for timely decision-making.
- Automation: These sensors can be integrated with milking systems for automated sample collection, reducing labor requirements.
- Data-Driven Decisions: Continuous monitoring of progesterone levels can help farmers make informed decisions about breeding management and reproductive interventions.

## Challenges and Considerations

- Sensor Calibration and Accuracy: Sensors need to be properly calibrated to ensure accurate progesterone measurements.
- Sensor Maintenance: Regular maintenance and quality control are necessary to ensure reliable and consistent results.
- Herd Variability: Individual animals may have varying baseline progesterone levels, and sensor data should be interpreted in the context of the specific herd's characteristics.
- Milk progesterone sensors are a valuable tool for improving reproductive management in farm animals. However, successful implementation requires proper training, quality control procedures, and an understanding of the specific reproductive physiology of the animals being monitored.

## Pregnancy-associated glycoproteins (PAGs) based pregnancy diagnosis

Pregnancy-associated glycoproteins (PAGs). The translocation of extraembryonic trophoblastic cell layers into the endometrium between days 20 and 28 and the secretions of the conceptus lead to successful implantation and continuation of pregnancy in ruminants. Pregnancy-associated glycoproteins (PAGs) are secretion products of mononuclear and binucleate trophoblast cells in bovine placenta. Among these glycoproteins, two pregnancy-specific proteins in the sera of pregnant cows, a 65–70kDa and a 47–53kDa protein with a pI of 4.6 – 4.8 and 4.0 – 4.4, respectively. Of these, the former showed an immune response similar to that of α 1-fetoprotein, while the latter showed no reactivity with known proteins and was given the name "protein B" or "pregnancy-specific protein B" (PSPB) in cattle.

Further purification and characterization of several isoforms from foetal bovine cotyledons revealed that protein B is indeed a 67-kDa PAG. Biochemical and functional studies revealed that these proteins are enzymatically inactive members of the superfamily of asparagine proteinases that share homology with pepsin, chymosin, cathepsin D, and the enzyme renin.

PAGs are a very complex group of proteins, as evidenced by the 22 different cDNA libraries already documented. The three best studied bovine PAGs, PSPB, PAG 67 kDa or bPAG-1, and PSP60, are isomers of the same protein with similar N-terminal sequences. Transcription of the mRNA of bPAG-2 and -11 occurs throughout gestation; the mRNA of -4, -5, and -9 in early gestation and the mRNA of bPAG-1 are not detectable until after day 45. Interestingly, bovine PAG-4 and bPAG-1 mRNA are highly transcribed by day 250 of gestation but are undetectable by the end of gestation. The six N-glycosylation sites are responsible for the variations in molecular weight and half-life of PAGs and are also the reason for the expression of different PAGs during different stages of gestation. Recently, it has been observed that placental defects, which frequently occur during somatic nuclear transfer in cattle, are complemented by abnormally high plasma levels of PAGs, probably due to decreased clearance of these proteins as a result of changes in glycosylation patterns. PSPB is detectable in the serum of pregnant cows over a long period of gestation, beginning around the fourth week of gestation and continuing until several weeks after parturition. High circulating concentrations of these proteins on days 80 to 100 postpartum limit their use as a pregnancy diagnostic test, except in heifers.

Sasser and co-workers developed a two- antibody radioimmunoassay for serological detection of PSPB for pregnancy diagnosis in cattle and found that serum levels increased from 1 ng/mL after day 30 to 9 ng/mL, 35ng/mL and 150ng/mL at three, six and nine months of gestation, respectively. The study claimed that PSPB detection is more accurate than the traditional rectal palpation method for detecting pregnancy. A sandwich ELISA using anti-PAG monoclonal antibodies has been developed that detected PAG in all pregnant animals, with concentrations of 8.75 ng/mL at day 28, the highest value of 588.9 ng/mL at the week of parturition, and very low values within four weeks of parturition. Several homologous (RIA -497) and heterologous radioimmunoassay systems (RIA -706, RIA -780, RIA -809, and RIA Pool) developed for measuring PAG concentrations in ruminant blood are highly correlated and can be used for pregnancy detection from 30–80 days. In radio-immuno-assays of pregnant sera from zebu cattle, PAG concentrations of 6.0 ng/ml, 196.0 ng/ml, 1095.6 ng/ml, and 348.4 ng/ml were detected at week 8, week 35, respectively. Results of PAG-RIA -based pregnancy diagnosis in buffalo are also encouraging, showing high diagnostic accuracy as early as day 31, with sensitivity of 100% and specificity of 90–100%. PAGs are being used to develop bench-top pregnancy detection assays that are now commercially available as BioPRYN (BioTracking, Russia), DG29 (Genex Cooperative Inc., USA), and IDEXX (IDEXX Laboratories, Inc., USA). The BioPRYN blood test is the most widely used PAG-based kit for pregnancy detection in ruminants.

## Preg – D®: Urinemetabolite-based Pregnancy Diagnosis

Preg D is a patented (Indian patent "Urine-based pregnancy detection method for ruminants", filed under No. 202011013074, dated March 25, 2020) urine-based pregnancy detection kit for use in cattle and buffaloes, developed by ICAR-Central Institute for Research on Buffaloes, Hisar

## About the Technology

The Preg-D kit is a novel urine-based method for pregnancy diagnosis in dairy animals. The kit uses a simple thermophilic biochemical colour reaction in urine for pregnancy diagnosis and can be performed by any educated person. No instruments are required to read the results - interpretation is done by observing the colour development. The kit is a very effective alternative method for identifying non-pregnant animals in the herd. The kit can be used by the farmer himself, which is very useful in rural areas where it is very difficult to find a veterinarian for pregnancy diagnosis.

The method is based on a colorimetric assay of at least six metabolites that form a red-purple coloured lactone derivative conjugate [(2,5-dihydro-4-methyl-5-(2,6,6-trimethyl-4-oxocyclohex-2-enylmethylene) furan-2-one called the Preg-D Pregnancy Diagnostic Kit for Cattle. The colour intensity is highest around day 150 until the end of pregnancy, which was confirmed by measuring the intensity at a wavelength of 665 nm. A patent has been filed for the developed method (see Indian patent "Urine based pregnancy detection method for ruminant livestock animals", filed under number 202011013074, dated March 25, 2020)

The method and kit are suitable for pregnancy diagnosis after completion of the oestrus cycle in cows/buffaloes. Considering that the biological process of pregnancy detection in cattle is completed around day 40 after insemination, the method (and thus the kit) provides high accuracy around days 30-40 of gestation. However, the test is sensitive and can detect pregnancy in most animals as early as day 18. To obtain more accurate results, the test should be repeated after 12-15 days.

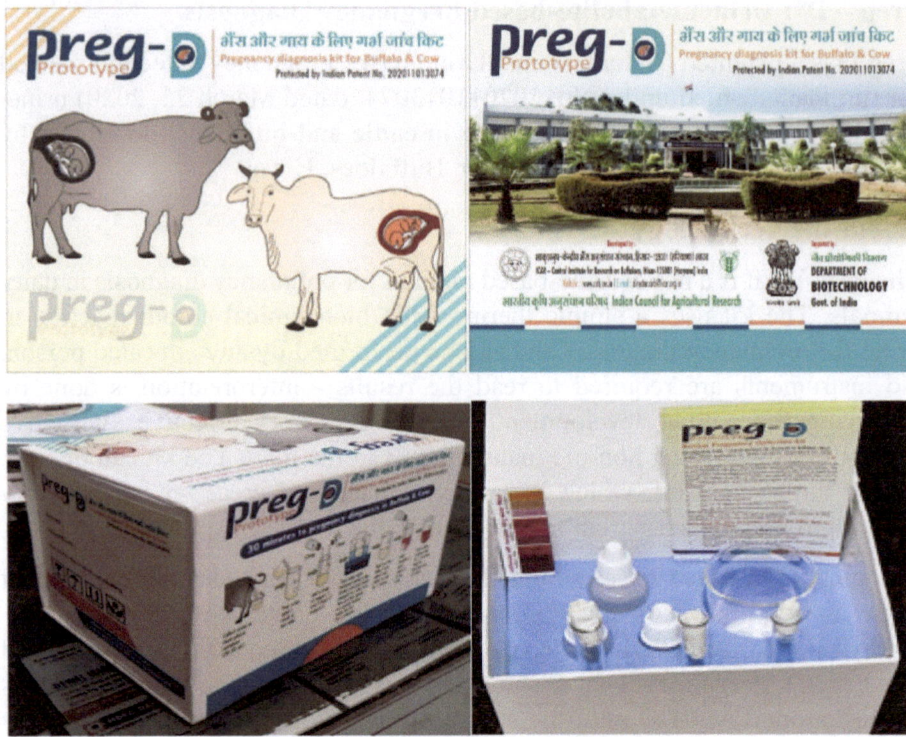


**Figure 4:** Preg- D bovine pregnancy diagnosis kit

This kit is intended for pregnancy testing after completion of the oestrus cycle in cows/buffalo (30 days after artificial insemination/natural mating). The test is sensitive and can detect pregnancy in most animals as early as day 18. For more accurate results, the test should be repeated after 12-15 days. As pregnancy progresses, there is increased secretion of metabolites that cause a color reaction. By day 150 of gestation, the color intensity of these metabolites is maximal and remains high until calving.

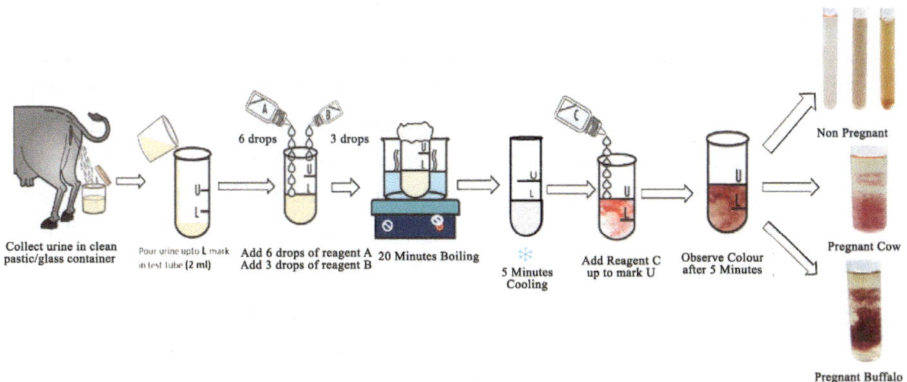


**Figure 5:** Performing pregnancy diagnosis using Preg D kit

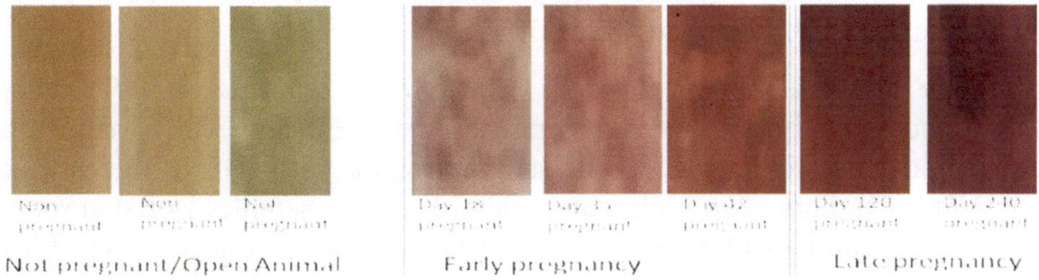


**Figure 6:** Colour patterns for identifying pregnancy in bovine species

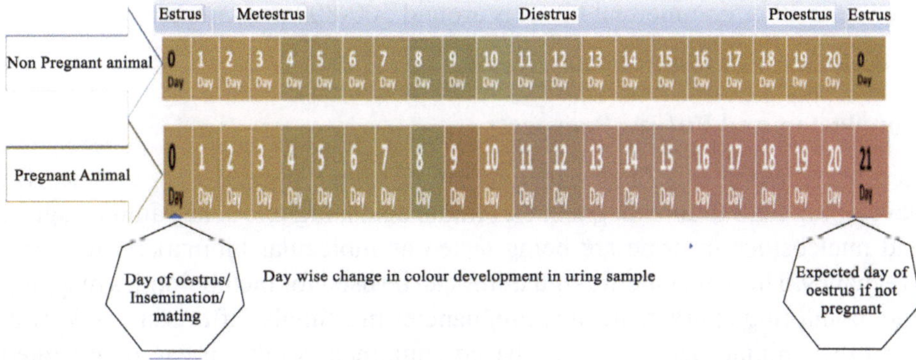


**Figure 7:** Colour variation with progression of pregnancy

## Advantages of using Preg D over other test kits

1. ***Ease of use:*** Preg D is perhaps the only urine-based pregnancy diagnostic kit. To date, there are no field-ready urine-based pregnancy diagnostic kits for dairy buffalo and cows. From time to time, some progesterone-based kits have appeared, but their accuracy is always questionable. Urine collection from animals does not require physical restraint/surgery with surgical equipment. Therefore, urine-based tests are considered non-invasive methods.

   Since the test kit is based on urine, the animal is not injured during sample collection, making it a non-invasive method. Kits based on blood require physically restraining the animal in a chute and drawing blood from a vein - an invasive method. The commercial kits (IDEXX, BIOPRYN, etc.) available for pregnancy diagnosis are based on PAGs and require blood to be drawn from the animal.

2. ***No cold chain/ refrigeration required for kit and sample:*** other commercially available kits are based on ELISA, which require a cold chain for storage of the sample and the kit itself. In the case of Preg-D, there is no such requirement, i.e. urine samples stored at room temperature can be processed up to 12 hours after collection. The kit's reagents also do not need to be stored at cold temperatures.

3. ***Cost effective*** – Per sample testing using Preg D comes around 5-10 Rs. For other commercial kits it is around 500-800 per sample.

4. Reading of results by naked eye

## Conclusion and Future Prospects

Recent developments in urinary metabolites have opened new avenues for developing field usable diagnostics. Amino acids, organic acids, amino sugars, and nucleosides in urine are being tested as molecular biomarkers for early pregnancy. These metabolite signatures can be used for metabolomics mapping and monitoring to assess healthy pregnancies in animals. Efforts are underway to further miniaturize the sensor-based equipment so that it can be operated under all types of field conditions.

## Suggested Readings

Balhara AK, Gupta M, Singh S, Mohanty AK and Singh I (2013) Early Pregnancy Diagnosis in Bovines: Current Status and Future Directions. The Scientific World Journal. Published online Article ID 958540, 10 pages, doi:10.1155/2013/958540

Bathla, S., Rawat, P., Baithalu, R., Yadav, M. L., Naru, J., Tiwari, A., Balhara, A. K., ... & Mohanty, A. K. (2015). Profiling of urinary proteins in Karan Fries cows reveals more than 1550 proteins. Journal of proteomics, 127, 193-201.

Sarangi, A., Ghosh, M., Sangwan, S., Kumar, R., Balhara, S., Phulia, S. K., ... &Balhara, A. K. (2022). Exploration of urinary metabolite dynamicity for early detection of pregnancy in water buffaloes. Scientific Reports, 12(1), 16295.

Zhou, C., Cai, G., Meng, F., Hu, Q., Liang, G., Gu, T., . & Hong, L. (2022). Urinary metabolomics reveals the biological characteristics of early pregnancy in pigs. Porcine Health Management, 8(1), 1-12.

# 6

# Reproductive Management for Augmenting Fertility at Dairy Farms

***Navdeep Singh***

*Directorate of Livestock Farms, Guru Angad Dev Veterinary and Animal Sciences University, Ludhiana, Punjab*

## Abstract

*Reproductive challenges in bovine dairy farming, including reduced conception rates and extended calving intervals, pose significant obstacles to industry productivity and genetic advancement. This article advocates for a comprehensive strategy that addresses these challenges through the integration of effective reproductive management, nutritional optimization, advanced technologies, and robust biosecurity measures.Meticulous record-keeping emerges as a fundamental element, providing insights into high-performing animals and facilitating strategic culling of those facing reproductive challenges. Efficient oestrus detection is highlighted, with precision dairy farming sensors offering real-time insights into oestrous cycles. The article emphasizes proper artificial insemination techniques, semen handling, and the incorporation of ultrasonography for early pregnancy diagnosis, contributing to enhanced reproductive outcomes.The intricate interplay between nutrition and reproduction is explored, emphasizing the importance of balanced energy, protein, fats, minerals, and vitamins. Heat stress, a notable factor influencing bovine reproduction, is mitigated through pre- and post-artificial insemination cooling strategies. Farm biosecurity measures, encompassing strict quarantine practices and disease surveillance, play a pivotal role in preventing infectious diseases and supporting overall herd health. This holistic approach aims to synergize various strategies, enhancing reproductive efficiency, safeguarding herd health, and promoting the overall productivity and sustainability of the cattle and buffalo industries. The proposed comprehensive strategy seeks to yield healthier cows, improved productivity, and sustained success in the dynamic landscape of dairy farming.*

**Keywords:** Reproductive efficiency, Bovine dairy farming, Conception rate, Nutritional optimization, Precision dairy farming.

Reproductive problems in bovine dairy farms can significantly impact the productivity and sustainability of the cattle and buffalo industry. Challenges such as diminished conception rates, delayed age at first calving, prolonged calving intervals, and higher embryonic losses have comprehensive implications, resulting in economic setbacks and impeding genetic advancements. These intricate problems are attributed to a combination of factors encompassing deficient reproductive management strategies, inadequate nutritional provisions, suboptimal breeding methodologies, the prevalence of infectious diseases, and the impact of environmental stressors. Inadequate management of the estrus cycle and mistimed insemination practices underscore the significance of effective reproductive management. Poor nutritional support can detrimentally affect the onset of puberty, compromise the quality of oocytes and embryos, and usher in an overall decline in reproductive performance. The presence of infectious diseases not only intensifies difficulties in achieving successful conception but also amplifies the rates of embryonic as well as pregnancy loss.

Additionally, environmental stressors, particularly heat stress, can disrupt estrus patterns, impede oocyte development, and hinder embryo growth. Consequently, addressing these complex reproductive issues necessitates a comprehensive and multifaceted approach. This approach entails the implementation of sound reproductive management protocols to ensure precise monitoring of estrus cycles and timely insemination practices through proper record-keeping. Furthermore, optimizing nutritional provisions tailored to distinct reproductive stages enhances ovarian function, augments oocyte quality, and promotes healthy embryo development. Rigorous biosecurity measures, including strict quarantine practices and adherence to vaccination regimens, play a pivotal role in disease prevention and control within the farm environment. Moreover, the integration of advanced reproductive technologies, such as ultrasonography and embryo transfer, offers avenues for early pregnancy detection and facilitates selective breeding to enhance genetic progress. By amalgamating these strategies, a concerted effort can be made to enhance reproductive efficiency, safeguard herd health, and ultimately support the overall productivity and sustainability of the cattle and buffalo industries.

## Reproductive Management

### *Record keeping*

Record keeping stands as a cornerstone for achieving optimal reproductive efficiency within dairy farming operations. The foundation of effective record keeping lies in meticulous maintenance of individual animal records spanning from birth to sale or demise. These records include a comprehensive reproductive history, encompassing crucial details such as oestrous cycles, insemination occurrences, pregnancy diagnosis dates, and calving dates. Additionally, any medicinal or hormonal interventions administered throughout the animal's lifecycle should be diligently documented. The power of these records lies in the insights they yield. By scrutinizing the collected data, animals exhibiting favourable reproductive performance metrics such as low age at first calving (AFC) and lower calving intervals can be identified. These insights empower farmers to make informed decisions when it comes to selecting breeding candidates that are likely to contribute to a healthy and productive herd. Furthermore, record keeping shows a dual advantage. Animals that face reproductive challenges, especially when juxtaposed with milk production performance, can be systematically culled from the herd. This strategic culling not only ensures the perpetuation of a robust breeding program but also contributed to efficient resource allocation. In essence, record keeping serves as the compass guiding dairy farmers towards informed and strategic reproductive management. The ability to discern patterns, identify outliers, and align breeding decisions with performance data translates into enhanced herd health, improves reproductive outcomes, and ultimately, a more sustainable and prosperous dairy farming venture.

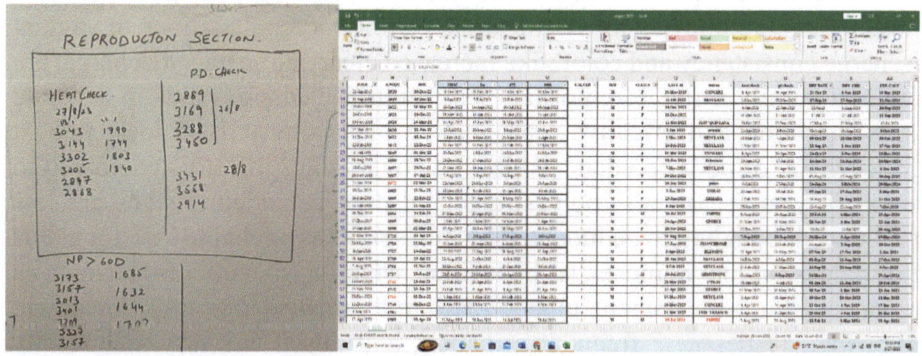


**Figure 1.** Heat expectancy charts excel sheet records.

***Efficient Estrus detection:*** Estrus, a pivotal phase in the reproductive cycle of female animals, marks the period during which they become sexually receptive. The unmistakable sign of a cow standing to be mounted by bull or other cows signifies estrus. However, this phenomenon is less conspicuous in buffaloes compared to cattle. As buffaloes and cattle form the cornerstone of India's milk production, primarily in rural areas, effective management practices are essential to enhance their productivity. These practices aid in identifying estrus in both cattle and buffaloes. Notably, a majority of these animals exhibit peak sexual activity during late evenings or early mornings, emphasizing the importance of deploying extra labor or providing incentives to supervisors and animal attendants to identify estrus events.

After the end of estrus, which typically lasts for 12 to 18 hours but can vary from 4 to 24 hours, ovulation occurs around 10-12 hours later. The estrous cycle accomplices the hormonal and reproductive challenges occurring from one heat period to the next. While the average length of estrous cycle is 21 days, it may vary between 17 to 24 days. The significance of detecting estrus lies in its potential to improve reproductive efficiency, shorten calving intervals, and enhanced conception rates.

Estrus signs in cattle manifest primarily as standing to be mounted, which is considered the most accurate indicator of estrus. Standing heat, the most sexually intense period of the estrous cycle, typically lasts for 15 to 18 hours but can vary from 8 to 30 hours. A cow in estrous usually stands to be mounted 22 to 55 times during her estrus period, and each mount lasts 3-7 seconds. Secondary signs includes mounting other cows, mucus discharge, vulva swelling, bellowing, restlessness, and more. Furthermore, the research data reveals increased uterine tone during estrus, enhances uterine receptivity for potential embryo implantation. Ovaries exhibit follicular growth and ovulation, releasing mature oocytes for fertilization. Furthermore, alterations in vaginal discharge consistency and color, like increased clear and stringy discharge, are common during estrus. Monitoring these multifaceted signs aids in accurate estrus detection and effective reproductive management Buffaloes, known for being shy or poor breeders, exhibit less overt signs of estrus compared to cattle. They are seasonally polyestrous, and their behavioural signs are less pronounced. Standing to be mounted by bull serves as a reliable sign for estrus in buffaloes, unlike homosexual behaviour, which is sporadic. Signs such as vulvar swelling, transparent mucus discharge, spontaneous milk let down, bellowing,, restlessness frequent urination, and raised tail vary in intensity among animals.

Various methods are employed to detect estrus in cattle and buffaloes. Physical methods involve visual and personal observations, sound record keeping, heat expectancy charts, vaginal probes, pedometers, tail paints, gimbal markers, teaser bulls, and advanced technologies such as CCTV camera or heat watch systems. Biological methods for estrus detection involve trained dogs and teaser bulls, including vasectomized bull, androgenized steers and surgical diverted penises.

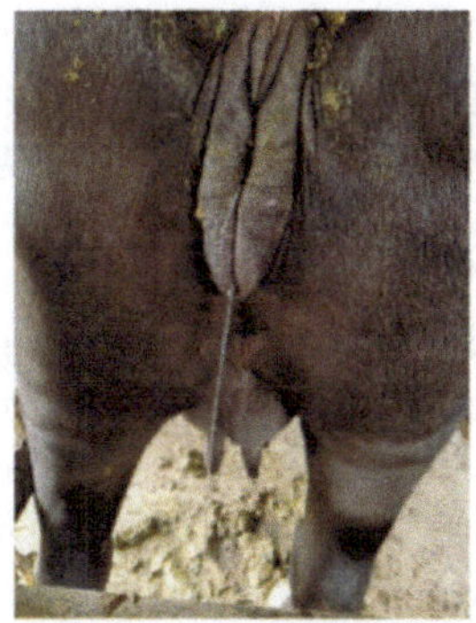

**Figure 2:** Clear and stringy discharge

Use of precision dairy farming sensors: Precision dairy farming has embraced advanced sensor technologies to enhance heat detection and health monitoring in cattle. These sensors offer real- time insights to individual animal's behavior, enabling accurate identification of estrus cycles based on increased activity and mounting events. Additionally, they monitor vital signs and detect deviations in temperature, rumination, and minimizing the impact of diseases. By using precision farming sensors, dairy operation can improve reproductive efficiency and overall herd well-being, leading to higher productivity and sustainability.

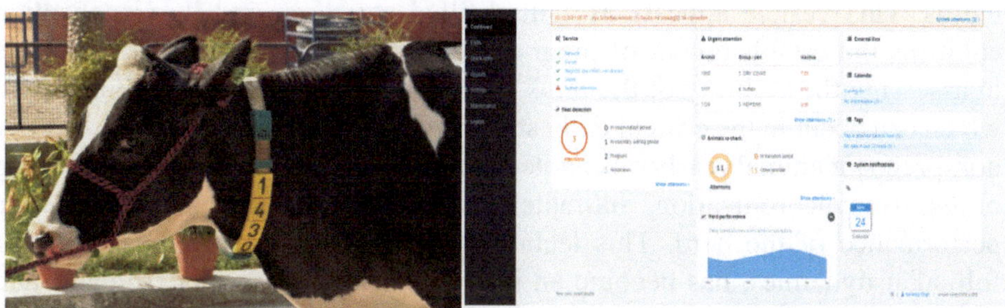

**Figure 3:** Precision dairy sensors

## Proper Artificial insemination techniques and semen handling

Proper artificial insemination (AI) techniques, along with meticulous semen thawing protocols, have been demonstrated to play a crucial role in enhancing reproductive outcomes in both cattle and buffalo farming. In cattle, AI has revolutionized breeding practices, allowing the utilization of genetically superior sires to propagate desirable traits. Research indicates that proficient AI practices have led to impressive conception rates, ranging from 50% to 75% in dairy cattle. It is worth noting that the correct thawing of frozen semen is equally vital. Studies reveal that employing standardized thawing methods yields improved results, with post-thaw motility rates of about 40% to 60% in cattle. Buffalo farming similarly benefits from the implementation of proper AI and semen thawing techniques. AI has been a pivotal factor in enhancing buffalo genetics, productivity, and disease management. Effective AI practices have resulted in notable conception rates of around 50% to 60% in buffaloes, contributing significantly to the overall improvement of herd quality. Ensuring accurate semen thawing procedures is vital for maintaining optimal sperm viability. Research findings suggest that thawing buffalo semen at 37°C for 30 to 40 seconds can result in post-thaw motility rates of approximately 40% to 50%. The successful implementation of these techniques not only enhances reproductive efficiency but also plays a pivotal role in ensuring the sustainable development of livestock industries.

## Use of Ultrasonography at Farms

The use of ultrasonography has revolutionized early pregnancy diagnosis in bovine reproduction, significantly contributing to the improvement of reproductive efficiency on farms. Ultrasonography allows veterinarians and farmers to detect pregnancies as early as day 28 after breeding, providing a substantial advantage over traditional methods. One crucial indicator observed through ultrasonography is the presence of an embryonic vesicle within the uterus. This vesicle appears as a fluid-filled structure, and its visualization confirms the establishment of pregnancy. Additionally, ultrasonography aids in assessing the viability of the fetus and identifying cases of embryonic loss, which can occur in the critical early stages of pregnancy. The ability to identify non-pregnant animals early on enables timely intervention, such as re-breeding or estrus synchronization, ultimately enhancing the overall reproductive performance of the herd. This technology, coupled with the monitoring of follicular dynamics, has become an indispensable tool for modern dairy and beef operations, ensuring efficient reproductive management.

## Impact of Nutrition on Reproductive Efficiency of Farms

The intricate interplay between nutrition and reproduction is a cornerstone of dairy cattle management, garnering increasing attention from producers, veterinarians, and researchers alike. Recognizing and understanding the profound connection between these two factors is pivotal for achieving optimal reproductive performance and enhancing overall herd health. This intricate relationship encompasses various dimensions, ranging from the impact of nutrition on ovarian function and embryo development to its influence on conception rates and the critical transition period.

***Energy**:* The importance of energy intake cannot be overstated in maintaining robust reproductive performance. Insufficient energy supply can lead to delayed puberty, extended intervals from parturition to conception, and disrupted ovarian cyclicity. When energy is prioritized for basic metabolic functions, growth, and lactation, reproductive processes may be compromised, resulting in decreased fertility rates. Thus, meticulous management of energy intake during late gestation and postpartum phases is pivotal for preserving optimal reproductive function.

***Protein**:* Dietary protein levels exert a multifaceted influence on reproductive function. Both inadequate and excessive protein intake can have adverse effects on reproduction. Overfeeding degradable intake protein (DIP), which includes protein and urea, has been linked to decreased pregnancy rates in female cattle. High levels of ammonia or urea exposure may hinder oocyte maturation and embryonic development. Striking the right balance between providing sufficient protein while avoiding overfeeding is crucial to maintaining optimal fertility.

***Fats and Hormones:*** Dietary fats and cholesterol play a vital role in hormone synthesis, potentially affecting reproductive hormone levels and the overall reproductive axis. Diets rich in fatty acids can enhance progesterone production and extend the lifespan of the corpus luteum (CL), ultimately boosting fertility. With proper management, high-fat diets can promote positive reproductive outcomes by stimulating progesterone levels during the luteal phase and fostering follicular growth.

***Minerals**:* Essential minerals, such as phosphorus, calcium, selenium, zinc, copper, iodine, and magnesium, are integral to reproductive processes. Insufficient or imbalanced mineral intake can negatively impact reproductive outcomes. The dietary cation-anion difference (DCAD), encompassing sodium, potassium, chloride, and sulphur levels, holds particular significance during the transition period. Maintaining a negative DCAD before calving helps prevent postpartum metabolic disorders and supports successful early lactation.

***Vitamins:*** Vitamins play a crucial role in reproduction. Vitamin A, for instance, influences ovarian follicular growth, uterine environments, and oocyte maturation. Adequate vitamin D is essential for proper calcium and phosphorus metabolism, while vitamin E functions as an antioxidant, safeguarding cellular integrity against oxidative damage. Ensuring appropriate vitamin and mineral supplementation, particularly in environments with limited natural sunlight, contributes to optimal reproductive health.

## Transition Period Management

Managing transition cows effectively is paramount for ensuring favourable reproductive outcomes and overall health. This critical period, spanning roughly three weeks before and after parturition, marks a pivotal phase in the lifecycle of lactating cows. A convergence of factors makes these cows particularly susceptible to metabolic and infectious diseases, including mastitis and metritis. The rapid increase in fetal demands and the concurrent development of the mammary gland trigger profound adaptive changes at physiological, metabolic, and nutritional levels, defining the transition from gestation to lactation.

Challenges during this period include reduced dry matter intake, often leading to the mobilization of adipose tissue reserves. While cows can often manage this physiological response, excessive metabolic demands can lead to health issues. This underscores the importance of addressing Negative Energy Balance (NEB), where the energy required for milk synthesis and secretion exceeds available energy from feed. Excessive NEB compromises immune systems and overall well-being, rendering cows susceptible to diseases. The immune system of cows under metabolic stress becomes compromised, highlighting the intricate link between metabolic status and peripartum immune function. To mitigate the impacts of NEB and associated metabolic challenges, providing adequate nutritional support post-calving is essential. This is especially vital as peak lactation energy demands can lead to substantial negative energy balance.

Negative energy balance also negatively affects fertility. Reduced dry matter intake post-calving can delay ovulation, leading to postponed conception. Altered concentrations of hormones such as insulin, glucose, growth hormone, and non-esterified fatty acids (NEFAs) disrupt the intricate hypothalamic-pituitary-gonadal (HPG) axis, contributing to postpartum infertility. Pre-calving loss of body condition further accentuates these effects, culminating in delayed postpartum ovarian rebound and compromised reproductive function.

Ovarian follicles are key players in this interplay, as they house insulin receptors. Lower peripheral insulin levels postpartum can delay ovarian resumption and cyclicity and increase the risk of cystic ovarian disease. Dietary interventions that enhance peripheral insulin concentrations postpartum play a pivotal role in restoring normal ovarian function. Dietary fats, particularly those with glucogenic properties, contribute by restoring energy balance and influencing cellular functions affecting ovarian and uterine health.

To address challenges posed by negative energy balance, researchers have explored various strategies. Incorporating bypass fats into diets has shown promise, influencing gene expression crucial to reproductive events and steroidal hormone synthesis. Additionally, dietary fats impact cholesterol circulation, a precursor to hormones like progesterone. These interventions restore energy balance and regulate pathways influencing reproductive health.

Antioxidants have also emerged as valuable tools for promoting fertility during the transition period. Oxidative stress, resulting from an imbalance between reactive oxygen species and the body's ability to neutralize them, affects various reproductive stages. Incorporating antioxidant-rich diets and herbal supplements mitigates oxidative stress and its damaging effects on reproduction. Plant-based compounds and formulations with potent antioxidant properties are gaining attention for their potential benefits.

## Optimizing Reproductive Efficiency with Managed Breeding Programs and Estrous/Ovulation Synchronization

Extending the calving-to-conception interval beyond three months poses a significant risk of prolonged calving intervals and substantial economic losses in the dairy industry. The application of pharmaceutical interventions to regulate follicular, corpus luteum (CL), and uterine functions using prostaglandin (PGF), gonadotropin-releasing hormone (GnRH), and intravaginal progesterone-releasing inserts has paved the way for the development of highly effective timed-insemination protocols, particularly for first breeding attempts. However, the success of postovulatory increases in progesterone, which have the potential to boost pregnancy rates in specific groups of lactating dairy cows, relies on careful control of timing and dosing.

The introduction of controlled breeding protocols has made it feasible to induce estrus in postpartum anestrus animals with inactive ovaries. Diverse hormonal protocols have been devised to induce follicular growth, trigger luteolysis, and promote ovulation through fixed- time artificial insemination (FTAI), eliminating the need for observing estrus behavior. These protocols not only mitigate the risk of fertility losses due to errors in estrus detection but also emerge as strategic tools for enhancing conception rates and overall reproductive efficiency. Furthermore, resynchronizing non-responsive cows, coupled with the utilization of ultrasonography for early pregnancy diagnosis, provides the opportunity for a second timed-insemination within 3-5 days of a non-pregnant bovines.

Fundamental approaches to estrous synchronization involve either shortening the luteal phase through PGF injections or extending it using progesterone therapy. In both methods, vigilant estrus detection is essential for breeding responsive cases. The former approach includes two prostaglandin F2α injections spaced 11 days apart, followed by artificial insemination (AI) of animals detected in estrus within 4-5 days of the second PGF injection. However, this method is limited to animals with functional or persistent corpus luteum (CL), making it effective for cyclic animals' estrus synchronization but not for true anestrus cases. Conversely, the latter approach is versatile, serving both the purposes of estrus induction and synchronization. In this method, progesterone is administered (oral/subcutaneous/intramuscular/intravaginal) either for an extended period of 14-15 days (when used alone) or for a shorter period of 7-9 days (when combined with PGF at progesterone withdrawal).

Incorporating GnRH with basic synchronization methods facilitates ovulation synchronization, opening doors for FTAI in herds without substantial investments of time and labor in estrus detection. The foundational ovulation synchronization program, OvSynch protocol, involves GnRH injection (10 µg on day 0), PGF2α injection (500 µg on day 7), and a second GnRH injection (10 µg on day 9), followed by FTI 17-24 hours after the second GnRH injection. However, the initial service conception rate for a single round of OvSynch is approximately 30%, prompting diverse modifications to the basic protocol, such as preSynch, HeatSynch, doubleSynch, CoSynch, and Estra-doubleSynch, each with varying degrees of success. Progesterone-based programs (7-8 days' protocol) utilizing intravaginal devices with GnRH initiation and PGF termination (Day 7) have demonstrated improved synchronization and pregnancy rates in healthy cows compared to other methods.

## Heat Stress Impact on Reproductive Efficiency in Bovines

Heat stress exerts a significant impact on bovine reproduction, influencing conception rates and overall reproductive efficiency. Heat stress occurs when animals are unable to dissipate excess body heat effectively, and it has been well-documented that elevated environmental temperatures can lead to reduced reproductive performance in cattle. The Temperature-Humidity Index (THI) is commonly used to assess heat stress levels, with higher THI values indicating greater stress. Studies have shown that when THI exceeds a critical threshold, typically around 72-74, conception rates can decline substantially. High heat stress levels are associated with disrupted estrus cycles, decreased oocyte quality, and impaired embryo development, leading to a decreased likelihood of successful pregnancies.

To mitigate the adverse effects of heat stress on bovine reproduction, various management strategies are employed. One crucial approach is cooling the animals before and after artificial insemination (AI). Research has demonstrated that cooling cows before AI can significantly improve conception rates. Pre-AI cooling helps in reducing body temperature and alleviating the negative impacts of heat stress on reproductive processes. Additionally, cooling cows after AI is equally important, as high body temperature post-insemination has been linked to poor conception rates. Maintaining proper body temperature during this critical period is essential for successful embryo implantation and early pregnancy establishment.

Studies have shown that a mere one-degree increase in body temperature can result in decreased conception rates. Cattle are particularly vulnerable to heat stress due to their limited capacity to dissipate heat through sweating. When body temperature rises, it can disrupts ovulation, cause irregular estrus cycles, and even lead to embryonic mortality. Cooling strategies encompass providing shade, sprinklers, fans, and other cooling mechanisms to help cattle for maintaining comfortable body temperature. By addressing heat stress through effective cooling measures, dairy farmers can enhance reproductive performance and improve the overall health and productivity of their herds.

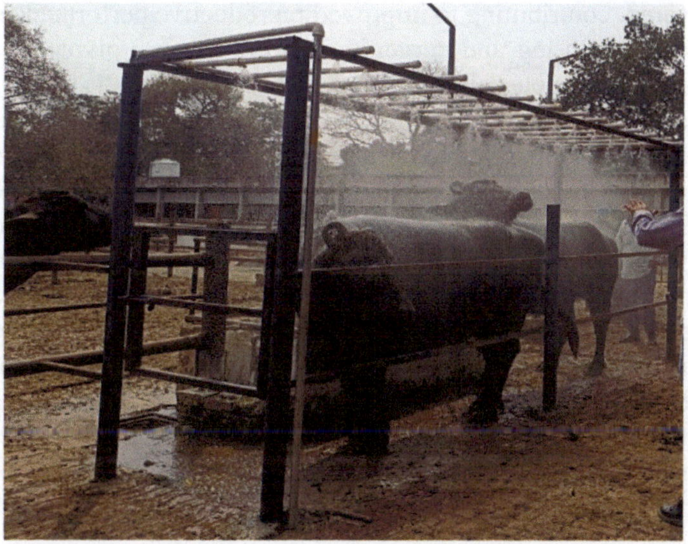

**Figure 4:** Cooling of animals before and after Artificial insemination

## Farm Biosecurity's Influence on Reproductive Efficiency in Dairy Farming

Disease control and farm biosecurity play integral roles in safeguarding the reproductive efficiency and overall health of dairy bovine herds. Biosecurity measures are a set of preventive practices implemented to minimize the introduction and spread of infectious agents within a herd, thus reducing the risk of disease outbreaks. A robust biosecurity plan encompasses various components that collectively contribute to optimizing reproductive outcomes and maintaining the well-being of the animals.

One of the key aspects of biosecurity is controlling the movement of animals, equipment, and personnel. Strict protocols for quarantine and isolation of incoming animals are essential to prevent the introduction of pathogens. New animals should undergo thorough health screenings and isolation periods to detect and address any potential disease carriers before they come into contact with the main herd. Additionally, limiting visitors and proper sanitation procedures upon entry reduces the risk of disease transmission. Maintaining a clean and hygienic environment is another crucial facet of biosecurity. Regular cleaning and disinfection of barns, equipment, and facilities can significantly curtail the survival and spread of infectious agents. Effective waste management, proper manure disposal, and prompt removal of carcasses further reduce disease vectors and reservoirs. By providing a clean-living space, the animals' stress levels are lowered, contributing to improved reproductive performance. Furthermore, disease monitoring and surveillance strategies are pivotal for early detection and prompt response. Regular health checks, diagnostic testing, and tracking of disease patterns enable timely interventions. Identification of potential carriers and carriers of specific reproductive pathogens, such as brucella abortus, bovine viral diarrhea virus (BVDV) and infectious bovine rhinotracheitis (IBR), allows for targeted management strategies. Vaccination programs tailored to the specific disease challenges faced by the herd can significantly enhance immunity and reproductive success. Reproductive efficiency is intricately linked to the overall health and stress levels of the animals. Disease challenges can lead to metabolic stress, immune suppression, and disruptions in hormonal balance, all of which can adversely affect estrus cycles, conception rates, and pregnancy maintenance. For instance, the impact of uterine infections on conception rates is well-documented, as infections can interfere with embryo implantation and uterine involution.

Research underscores the connection between disease control, biosecurity, and reproductive efficiency. Studies have shown that improved biosecurity practices, such as isolating and testing incoming animals, contribute to lower disease prevalence and subsequently lead to better reproductive outcomes. Moreover, biosecurity measures aimed at reducing the transmission of specific pathogens, like BVDV, have been associated with higher conception rates and reduced embryonic losses in cattle herds. In conclusion, disease control and farm biosecurity are integral to promoting reproductive efficiency and sustaining a healthy dairy bovine herd. Implementing stringent biosecurity measures, including quarantine procedures, hygiene protocols, and disease surveillance, can effectively minimize the risk of disease introduction and spread. By reducing the incidence of infectious agents, stressors on the animals' health are minimized, directly impacting their reproductive performance. The synergy between disease control and reproductive health underscores the importance of a comprehensive biosecurity strategy that not only protects animal health but also bolsters the economic viability of dairy farming.

## Conclusion

In dairy farming, enhancing reproductive efficiency requires meticulous record-keeping, efficient estrus detection, and advanced breeding synchronization. Nutrition's role is paramount, with optimized energy, protein, fat, mineral, and vitamin intake vital for fertility. Proper transition management minimizes negative energy balance effects, while cooling strategies counter heat stress impacts. Farm biosecurity prevents disease spread, protecting overall herd health and reproductive success. These elements synergize for a comprehensive approach, yielding healthier cows, improved productivity, and sustained success in the dairy industry

## Suggested Readings

Baruselli, P. S., Visintin, J. A., &Trinca, L. A. (2001). Use of embryo transfer and artificial insemination in buffalo. Animal Reproduction Science, 68(3-4), 355-365.

Bisla.A., Yadav,V., Dutt, R., Singh, G., &Gahalot, S. C. (2018). Fertility Augmentation Approaches in Dairy Animals - A Review. International Journal of Current Microbiology and Applied Sciences, 7(2), 2995-3007.

Collier, R. J., Dahl, G. E., VanBaale, M. J., & Thatcher, W. W. (2006). Effects of cooling strategies on performance and physiology of lactating dairy cows during summer heat stress. Journal of Dairy Science, 89(7), 2679-2693.

Das, G. K., & Khan, F. A. (2010). Buffalo reproduction in Asia: recent developments and future perspectives. Italian Journal of Animal Science, 8(sup1), 350-366.

Das, G. K. and Khan, F. A. (2010). Summer anoestrus in buffalo—A review. Reproduction in Domestic Animals, 45, e483–94.

Dobson, H., & Smith, R. F. (2000). What is stress, and how does it affect reproduction? Animal Reproduction Science, 60-61, 743-752.

García-Ispierto, I, López-Gatius, F., Bech-Sabat, G., Santolaria, P., Yániz, J. L., Nogareda, C., De Rensis, F. & López-Béjar, M. (2007). Climate factors affecting conception rate of high producing dairy cows in northeastern Spain. Theriogenology, 67, 1379–1385.

Lopes, G., & Reynolds, J. (2014). The effect of environmental stressors on bovine reproduction. Tropical Animal Health and Production, 46(3), 427-435.

Lucy, M. C. (2001). Reproductive loss in high-producing dairy cattle: where will it end? Journal of Dairy Science, 84(E), e127-e136.

Moghaddam, A., Karimi, I. &Pooyanmehr, M. (2009). Effects of short-term cooling on pregnancy rate of dairy heifers under summer heat stress. Vetetrinary Research Communication, 33, 567–575.

Nandi, S., &Kamilya, I. S. (2014). Artificial insemination in water buffalo. The Indian Journal of Animal Sciences, 84(5), 501-505..

Parr, R.A. &Rorie, R.W., 2005. Follicular dynamics, timing of ovulation, and early pregnancy in beef cattle monitored by transrectal ultrasonography. Journal of Animal Science, 83(2), pp.343-353.

Pursley, J. R., Mee, M. O., &Wiltbank, M. C. (1995). Synchronization of ovulation in dairy cows using PGF2α and GnRH. Theriogenology, 44(7), 915-923.

Singh, J., Kumar, V., & Sharma, A. (2017). Artificial insemination in buffalo: An overview. Veterinary World, 10(6), 707-712.

# 7

# Recent Approaches in Diagnosis and Treatment of Bovine Mastitis

***Dhiraj Kumar Gupta***

*Department of Veterinary Medicine, College of Veterinary Science Guru Angad Dev Veterinary and Animal Sciences University, Ludhiana, Punjab*

## Abstract

*Mastitis is an inflammation of the mammary gland in response to injury for the purpose of destroying or neutralizing the infectious agents and to prepare the way for healing and return to normal function. The economic losses due to mastitis worldwide are huge. Diminished udder health has serious implications for milk production, leading to decreases in milk yield, milk quality and increases in somatic cell count (SCC). Approximately 70-80% of losses are due to subclinical mastitis. Presence of mastitis causative organisms and antibiotic residues in milk following therapy of mastitis poses a major threat to the consumer health. Mastitis results in increase in the somatic cell count (SCC) and bacterial load of milk. The high SCC has lipolytic effect on fat and there is increased tendency for rancidity of milk and milk products. Also, total bacterial count of more than 100 000 cfu/ml milk could release hydrolytic enzymes, which spoil the milk and milk products. Once mastitis is diagnosed the main challenge for the veterinarian or the producer is to treat the animals in such a way that it will not deteriorate and become an economic burden to the production system. Given the complexity of mastitis and the variability in treatment responses, a multifaceted approach that considers factors such as pathogen susceptibility, host immune status, and environmental conditions may be necessary for successful management. Several therapeutic strategies like antibiotics, vaccines, bacteriocins, herbal therapy, immunotherapy, and nanoparticle technology have been evaluated for efficacy in treating mastitis, but no single technique was found to be effective in controlling or treating the disease due to the variable response of etiological agents to the therapeutic techniques.*

**Keywords:** Mastitis, SCC, Diagnosis, Treatment and prevention

Mastitis is a consequence of interplay between the infectious agents and managerial practices. The mammary glands of cows are frequently exposed to potential pathogens, but on most of the occasion, cows get mastitis because their immune systems are not adequate to prevent infection. Mastitis is an inflammation of the mammary gland in response to injury for the purpose of destroying or neutralizing the infectious agents and to prepare the way for healing and return to normal function. The average incidence of subclinical mastitis has been found to be 49% in cows and 28% in buffaloes. Similarly, clinical mastitis is prevalent in 7% of cows and 4% buffaloes. Besides this, 17% of the cows and 8% of buffaloes have been suffering from various udder and teat lesions such as udder/teat warts, bovine ulcerative mammilitis, udder impetigo and teat chaps etc. These lesions pre-dispose the animal to mastitis and cause a great discomfort at milking and hence markedly decrease the milk yield. The economic losses due to mastitis worldwide have been estimated at $35 billion. Current annual economic losses due to mastitis in India have been estimated to be Rs. 7165.51 crore that include Rs. 4151.16 crore and Rs. 3014.35 crore due to subclinical and clinical mastitis, respectively. Mastitis causes a reduced milk production, not only at its occurrence but throughout the rest of the lactation, increases the risk of new cases of mastitis and increases the risk of culling. Besides, mastitis impairs the quality of milk and milk products. Approximately 70-80% of losses are due to subclinical mastitis. Subclinical mastitis is also important due to the fact that it is 15-40 times more prevalent than the clinical form. It usually precedes the clinical form, is of longer duration, difficult to detect and constitutes a reservoir of micro-organisms that lead to infection of other animals within the herd.Besides this, presence of mastitis causative organisms and antibiotic residues in milk following therapy of mastitis poses a major threat to the consumer health. Mastitis results in increase in the somatic cell count (SCC) and bacterial load of milk. The European Union has set up a threshold of 400,0000 cells/ml of milk from healthy quarter of a cow. The high SCC in mastitis milk has lipolytic effect on fat and there is increased tendency for rancidity of milk and milk products. Also, the mastitis milk with total bacterial count of more than 100,000 cfu/ml could release hydrolytic enzymes, which spoil the milk and milk products. It has been also observed that mastitis milk inhibits the growth of starter bacteria and results in decreased cheese production.

- **Etiology of Disease Host adapted**
  - Mammary gland reservoir
  - Transmitted at milking
  - *S. aureus*, *S. agalactiae*, *Mycoplasma* spp.

- **Environmental**
  - Reservoir: environment
  - Transmission: between milkings
  - *E. coli, S. uberis,* other coliforms, *Pseudomonas*
- **Opportunists**
  - *S. dysgalactiae*
  - Non-aureus staphylococci
- **Other pathogens**
  - *S. zooepidemicus, S. fecalis, M. bovis, B. abortus*
  - *Trichosporon* spp., *Aspergillus* spp., *Candida* spp.
  - Trauma, chemical irritant, viral

## Diagnosis of Mastitis

In its clinical form, disease may be diagnosed well by the classical signs of inflammation and visible alterations in milk consistency, colour and appearance etc. The changes in levels at which certain components in the mammary secretion are present are commonly employed in identifying the disease at its subclinical level. A variety of diagnostic tests for mastitis are available which differ markedly with respect to sensitivity, specificity, simplicity, rapidity and cost. Among these, Bromothymol blue (BTB) card, Sodium lauryl sulphate (modified California mastitis test) and Electrical conductivity tests are simple and economical tests that can be performed as cow-side tests at the field level.

***Bromothymol blue card test:*** It is based on the principle that in mastitis, the pH of milk rises due to entry of bicarbonate salts from blood into milk. Depending upon the health status of quarter and hence pH, the colour of the dye changes from yellow (normal) to greenish-yellow (+), green (++) and blue (+++) when a drop of quarter milk is placed on the card. But, this test has comparatively less sensitivity.

***Sodium Lauryl Sulphate (SLS) test:*** It is based on the principle that reagent ruptures somatic cell releasing cellular proteins (DNA) that results in gel formation, and depending upon the degree of gel formation the reaction is scored as 0, Trace, 1, 2 and 3. Thus, this test gives the indirect estimate of milk somatic cell count. This test could be used with high accuracy for estimation of milk SCC (r = 0.84).

***Electrical conductivity test (EC):*** The ions in milk conduct electricity, such that any change in concentration of ions is reflected as a change in conductivity. Dissociated, inorganic salts such as sodium, chloride and potassium are the main contributors to conductivity. The EC is moderately influenced by milk constituents such as protein and fat, which reduces the conductance of ions. The normal mean EC values were found much less in buffaloes (3.91 mS/cm) than in crossbred cattle (5.41 mS/cm). Also, the discrimination ability for EC to differentiate between healthy and mastitis quarters was found more in cattle (75. 54%) than in buffaloes (66.0%). In overall, based on mean values, it is found that there is difference in conductivity of 0.5 to 1.5 mS/cm between the healthy and mastitis quarters. The EC could be measured by digital conductivity meters, which are easily available in the market. Even, hand-held battery-operated digital conductivity meters are available for use as cow-side test.

***Culture sensitivity testing (CST) of milk:*** It is done to identify the causative organism and test its *in vitro* sensitivity to the drugs so as to advise rational therapy of mastitis.

## Ultrasonography of Teat, Udder and Supramammary Lymph Nodes

For the diagnosis of mastitis, milk culture and bacterial isolation has been considered the gold standard technique. This can be further supplemented with ultrasonography, a quick non-invasive method for the early diagnosis and visualization of changes in teat tissue and supramammary lymph nodes which otherwise, may be difficult to diagnose on physical examination. The popularity of real-time ultrasonography has tremendously increased in recent years as a diagnostic as well as a research tool in veterinary and animal science. It can be used like a helpful tool to diagnose pathological alterations of the udder such as inflammation, mucosal lesions, tissue proliferation, foreign bodies, milk stones, congenital changes, hematoma and abscess etc. The technique is noninvasive, relatively simple and effective, safe to both the subject and the operator, portable, and ultra-rapid, since the ultrasonic image facilitates immediate interpretation and diagnosis in most circumstances. For the timely and more economical detection of subclinical mastitis, it can be used to observe the changes in the udder and teat tissues. It has been observed that in cases of mastitis there are changes in teat and glandular tissue and supramammary lymph nodes which may be easily visualized using ultrasonography.

## Infrared Thermography (IRT)

Infrared thermography (IRT) is also gaining momentum as a technique of future for early diagnosis of mastitis with ease of applicability. All objects emit infrared radiation proportional to their temperature in accordance with Stefan-law. Using this law, a thermal camera is utilized which detects the infrared radiation and creates a pictorial representation based on the heat generated without exposing users to harmful radiation. IRT has been used in both the medicine and veterinary field for a long period; it may not be a confirmatory diagnostic tool although it very well can be used to detect the location of a lesion so long as it is on the surface of the animal. IRT involves not only studying the temperature of the location of interest but in the patterns of temperatures in the location of interest and the vicinity of the location would help in accurately diagnosing the disease in an easy, non-invasive technique that can be then supplemented with the required specific diagnostic tool.

## Treatment of Mastitis

*In vitro* testing of milk samples revealed that drug sensitivity pattern of mastitis organisms goes on changing from time to time and place to place or farm to farm. So, treatment should be given preferably based on culture and sensitivity test. In acute or per acute cases, there is no time for these tests, so the therapy in such cases is based on the past data of herd infection and sensitivity reports. However, before starting therapy in such cases, the milk sample should be invariably taken and put to culture sensitivity so that the therapy may be changed if needed in the light of sensitivity report. Moreover, it may also be made clear that there is no surety that *in vitro* sensitivity determination will correlate with the *in vivo* treatment results. For example, enrofloxacin that shows high *in vitro* sensitivity and is pharmacologically considered to distribute well in the udder clinically proved to be less efficacious against staphylococcal mastitis because of its inability to kill intracellular organisms. On the other hand, amino-glycosides (gentamicin and neomycin) that are considered to have poor distribution in the udder, *in vivo* proved very much effective in treatment of clinical mastitis. The organism involved in mastitis also affects the efficacy of treatment. Streptococci respond well, staphylococci less and coliforms are difficult to treat due to severe per acute reaction.

For improving treatment following considerations are worthwhile.

### 1. Location and Pathology of Causative Organism

a. *Streptococcus agalactiae* and *Streptococcus dysgalactiae*: milk and living epithelial cells.

b. *Staphylococcus aureus*, *Streptococcus uberis* and *Acanthobacteriumpyogenes*: deep tissues of gland.

c. Coliform organisms: simultaneous infection of udder and other body organs

## 2. Selection of Antibacterial Agent

Treatment of mastitis involves systemic antibiotics or intramammary infusions. Ideally systemically administered antibiotics must reach udder and should achieve minimum inhibitory concentration (MIC) in milk and parenchyma. Thus, pharmacologic agents which are non-ionoized, lipid soluble and have low protein binding are predicted to reach the target tissue more efficiently. Also, the concentrations gradient, which serves as driving force for drugs in to tissue and secretions, is a function of drug's total dose and frequency of administration. Thus higher dose rate or frequency, is the concentration gradient pushing the drug in to udder.

Distribution of antibiotics in udder post-intramammary administration

| Good | Moderate | Poor |
|---|---|---|
| Ampicillin | Benzyl Penicillin | Aminoglycosides |
| Amoxicillin | Cloxacillin | Polymixin |
| Penethamate | Cephoxazole | |
| Novobiocin | Cephalonium | |
| Erythromycin | Tetracyclines | |
| Nitrofurans | | |
| Tylosin | | |

## 3. Route of Administration

Selection of the route of antibacterial gent is not only important because of treatment cost but treatment success also. The route of treatment is governed by degree of severity of mastitis, infective agent involved and milk yield of the affected quarters. Accordingly, parentral therapy with or without intramammary infusion is preferred in acute clinical mastitis because of the simple reason of poor and uneven distribution of drug as a result of compressed and blocked duct system owing to inflammation. Intramammary route is accepted route of choice for subclinical and mastitis with local signs. However, Staphylococcal mastitis is an exception. This organism is tissue invader and is located in interstitial tissue, micro abscesses and intra-cisternally in neutrophils, macrophages and epithelial cells, therefore parentral therapy should be preferred. It is advantageous to combine systemic and local therapy in treating acute clinical non gangrenous *S. aureus* mastitis.

### 4. Duration of Therapy

A course of 5-days treatment produces higher bacteriological cure rates than 3-day course of treatment.

### 5. Severity of the infection

For taking specific therapy, clinical mastitis is generally divided into three forms viz., per acute, acute and chronic form.

**Peracute mastitis:** It is generally caused by coliforms and it occurs commonly around calving but may develop at any time during lactation. The disease is usually sudden in onset: the cow may appear normal at one milking and at the next milking shows pronounced signs including anorexia, rise of temperature, depression, shivering and rumen stasis. Inflammatory signs in the udder may be minimal at this time and swelling may be detectable only after the udder is milked out. Later, the quarter is swollen and hard, the teat may be thickened, oedematous, hot to touch and sensitive. In the early stages, the milk may appear normal or faintly watery. Subsequently it may be serous and contain tiny particles. In severe cases it may become blood tinged. Recommended therapy includes the following:

- Removal of bacteria, toxins and inflammatory exudates from the mammary gland by frequent milking and even oxytocin injections (20-30 IU I/M) may be given.
- Appropriate antibacterial therapy to start with systemic administration that may be later (after 12-24 h) supplemented with suitable intramammary infusion.
- Fluid therapy; dextrose saline solution (10-20 L in first hour, up to 60 L in severe cases) to restore vital body fluids, dilute toxins and counteract acidosis. Even 5% sodium bicarbonate (150-250 G) with first 3-5 L of fluid may be given.
- Systemic glucocorticoids, Dexamethasone @ 1-3 mg/kg IV or IM once or may be repeated after 8-12 hours.
- Calcium borogluconate 20% @ 500 ml IV to counteract hypocalcaemia induced by endotoxin. Administer with care as such therapy may have damaging effects on the heart in animals that are in shock.
- NSAIDs reduces pain and inflammation, and restores appetite.
- Antihistaminic drugs and multivitamins.

**Acute mastitis:** In this form there is no systemic reaction. Primarily changes are observed in milk, which may contain flacks, become watery or thick, and sometimes may contain blood. The udder may become swollen and hard. The line of treatment includes use of antibacterial drugs plus calcium and multivitamin therapy. The combination therapy i.e. intramammary plus parenteral works well than the alone parenteral or intramammary. The important recommendations in mastitis therapy are (i) Use antibacterial on need for recommended time i.e. at least for 5-days (ii) Use appropriate dose and dosing interval (iii) Stick to the recommended milk withdrawal times.

**Chronic mastitis:** A case is considered chronic when (i) there is formation of fibrotic cord inside teat canal (ii) there is thick pus discharge, not responding to treatment (iii) there is frequent reoccurrence of mastitis in the same quarter. The treatment/surgery of chronic mastitis is not rewarding. Rather such cases should be isolated from the milking herd or the affected quarter may be permanently dried-off by producing a chemical mastitis. Infusing 30-60 ml of 3% silver nitrate solution or 20 ml of 5% copper sulphate solution can do it. If a severe local reaction occurs, the quarter should be milked out and stripped frequently until the reaction subsides. If no reaction occurs, the quarter is stripped out 10-14 days later. Two infusions may be given.

Successful treatment of clinical mastitis depends on several factors: antimicrobial treatment, causal agent identification, parity, stage of lactation, history of previous SCC, clinical mastitis and other systemic diseases. However, the recent approaches used for treating mastitis involve the use of natural therapeutics could serve as an alternative to antibiotic therapy.

## Bacteriophage Therapy

Treatment of biofilm forming bacteria poses a great challenge due to their resistance against conventional antibiotics. In such instances, other modes of therapy have to be selected for successful elimination of the etiological agent. Bacteriophages are a group of viruses that have the ability to infect and kill bacteria. They have the inherent ability to target and destroy specific bacterium and also the capacity to replicate exponentially which makes them a potential candidate against pathogenic bacteria. The utilization of a phage cocktail instead of a single bacteriophage is preferred.

## Bacteriophage endolysins

Another potential therapeutic agent, called endolysins derived from the bacteriophages are effective against Gram-positive pathogens. They are the proteins that allow the phage to escape from the bacterial cell during the phage lytic cycle by degrading the peptidoglycan layer of bacterial cell wall. A novel bacteriophage-derived peptidase, $CHAP_K$ has been found an effective biocidal agent that can be used for the rapid disruption of biofilm-forming staphylococci. Some of the anti-staphylococcal peptidoglycan hydrolases include lysostaphin, LasA, ALE-1, broth lysate, CsCl, LytM, AtlA, AtlE, LysK, SAL-1, MV-L, ClyS, and LysH5.

## Antimicrobial Peptides

Antimicrobial peptides (AMPs) are new generation antibiotics that destroy invading microorganisms and have a major role in the innate immune mechanism. They have broad-spectrum activity against several Gram-positive and Gram-negative bacteria including some of the drug-resistant strains. AMPs produce synergism when used along with conventional antibiotics. The therapeutic application of AMPs is very much limited in the present scenario due to the short half-life, high production cost, enzymatic degradation, and cytotoxic effects on the eukaryotic cells. The β-defensins and bacteriocins (Nisin and Bovicin HC5)are examples of antimicrobial peptides.

## Probiotics

Lactic acid bacteria can provide protection against mastitis when they are used as feed supplements, teat dip, and intramammary inoculation due to their potent immunomodulatory activity. The lactic acid bacteria colonize the udder and prevent mastitis by forming a protective biofilm, which inhibits the growth of mastitis-causing pathogens. The gut microbiome and their metabolites play an important role in maintaining the health of dairy cow. Lipopolysaccharide (LPS) and short-chain fatty acids are the two major products of gut microbes.

## Herbal Therapy

Herbal therapy is a promising area in treatment of mastitis as no adverse effect is associated with it. Medicinal plants can be used as an alternative therapeutic option or as an adjunct agent in managing bovine mastitis. They can be used as an anti-bacterial, anti-inflammatory, and immunomodulatory agent for the treatment of mastitis. The anti-inflammatory and anti-bacterial effects of herbs have been utilized effectively in the treatment of bovine mastitis. Neem, Giloy, Ashwagandha, Tulsi, Haldi, Aloe vera, Kali Mirch, Harad, etc. have been used effectively in control of mastitis.

## Homeopathy

Homeopathy is an effective option in some cases of mastitis but not under all circumstances. The homeopathic remedies are of plant, mineral or animal origin, and are usually given to the patients in very high dilutions. These dilutions are claimed to be activated through a special dilution and shaking process called potentiation. WHO has recognized the value of homeopathy as one of the system of traditional medicine that could be integrated with conventional medicine to provide health care. As such similar to the antibiotics, homeopathy may show effectiveness against the particular microbes.

## Immunotherapy

Immunotherapy is an alternative, immunologically-based treatment for mastitis. Microbeads carrying specific antibodies to the mastitis causing bacteria, interleukins, *Saccharomyces cerevisae* yeast, and anti-recombinant *S. uberis* adhesion molecules have been tried as immunomodulators.

## Nanoparticle-based therapy

Nanoparticle technology is another area that is currently developing as a delivery technique for antimicrobial agents and other drugs. Different types of nanoparticles have already been evaluated for the treatment of mastitis with positive results. Nanoparticle formulations will enhance the uptake of active compound by phagocytes and thereby improving its antibacterial activity. Nanoparticle-based therapeutic techniques like liposomes, nanogels, polymeric nanoparticles, inorganic nanoparticles, and solid lipid nanoparticles are gaining popularity as excellent tools for managing mastitis.

## Stem Cell Therapy

The stem cells of bovine mammary epithelial cells play a major role in maintaining the udder health. Such stem/progenitor cells can be utilized for treating mastitis induced structural/cytological defects in the bovine udder. Mesenchymal stem cells have anti-bacterial activity due to the ability to produce certain factors that inhibit bacterial growth.

## Acoustic Pulse Therapy

Acoustic pulse therapy (APT) also known as shockwave therapy utilizes the hand-held instrument that produces pulsing pressure waves. Such waves penetrate through the deeper tissues and can break scar tissue of the chronic wounds leading to revascularization. This therapy though appears promising but further extensive including the involved infectious agent types studies are desired to standardize the therapy.

Even though there are several well-established treatment techniques along with a great number of emerging techniques, treatment of mastitis will always be a challenge to the clinician/veterinarian due to its broad spectrum of etiological factors along with the wide variety of clinical manifestations. Farmer's role and perception towards management of mastitis are very important.

## Control of Mastitis

The mastitis control program is multi-factorial and plays a significant role in reducing the incidence of new infection and shortening the duration of existing intra-mammary infection. It consists of cow factors as well as environment factors. The five major steps in mastitis control program are (1) udder hygiene and proper milking methods, (2) proper installation, function, and maintenance of milking equipment, (3) dry cow management and therapy, (4) appropriate therapy of mastitis cases during lactation and (5) culling chronically infected cows. Other factors in mastitis control are maintaining clean, dry and comfortable housing areas, maintaining udder health, good record keeping, regular monitoring of udder health status, maintenance of good biosecurity for contagious pathogens and review of mastitis control program at regular intervals. These hygienic milking techniques and control measures reduce bacterial dissemination, transmission, and consequent infection but they do not completely prevent infections from occurring. The important features of a successful mastitis control programme are:

### *a) Minimising the Source of Infection*

Infection can be prevented by maintaining optimal environmental and milking hygiene, segregation and prompt treatment of clinical mastitis cases, culling of carriers and drying off of chronically infected quarters. The adoption of hygienic measures depends upon the epidemiology of the causative organisms. For example, in case of contagious organisms, which are transmitted from one to another animal through the milking equipment and milker's hands, proper washing of udder, cleanliness of milker's hands/milking machine clusters in between each milking and post-milking teat dipping in germicidal solution will reduce the infection to a great extent. On the other hand, for the organisms that come from the environment e.g., to prevent coliforms mastitis animal environment should be kept clean by frequent removal of dung, proper drainage, and adequate milking and feeding space should be provided.

### *b) Elimination of Existing udder Infections*

It is achieved by *Dry therapy*. The dry therapy is done at the end of lactation (after last milking) with a long-acting antibiotic intramammary preparation that maintains effective drug concentration for 6-8 weeks i.e., throughout the dry period. It not only eliminates the subclinical infections of previous lactation but also prevents new IMI and increases the milk production by about 8-10%. In addition, it improves the milk quality at calving and prevents the occurrence of clinical mastitis cases during dry period and around calving. Now dry therapy preparations such as Spectramast-DC and Cepravinare available in India.

### *c) Prevention of New Intramammary Infections (IMI)*

It is achieved by *Post milking teat dipping*. The teats of all the lactating cows and dry cows (during first 10-14 days of dry period) are dipped regularly after -every milking in a germicidal solution. The recommended teat dips are

1. Iodine (0.5%) solution + Glycerine @ 15% of iodine solution
2. Chlorhexidine (0.5%) solution + Glycerine@ 06% of chlorhexidine solution

The iodine teat dip is found best as it also treats various types of teat lesions and injuries.

## Increasing the Udder Resistance to Mastitis

Future trends in mastitis control are aimed at increasing the immunity of udder to mastitis pathogens. This can be achieved by use of non-specific (*cytokines/ proper nutrition*) and specific (*vaccination*) immunomodulators.

**1. *Nutrition*:** Even slightest deficiencies of certain vitamins (Vit E, C, A and ß-carotene) and micro-nutrients (Cu, Se, Zn, Co) are reported to have detrimental impact on the efficient functioning of immune system. Vitamin A is involved in maintaining a functional epithelium that provides a physical barrier to the entrance of pathogens. ß-carotene also referred as pro-vitamin A enhances the immune function and disease resistance. Zinc supplementation prevents the infection by strengthening the skin and stratified epithelium (keratinocytes) of teat canal. The biological role of Cu is exerted through a number of Cu containing proteins including ceruloplasmin and superoxide dismutase (SOD). Similarly, vitamin E and the Se containing enzyme glutathione peroxidase (GSH-pX) also act as integral part of the antioxidant system. Studies have shown that supplementation of cows during dry period and around calving (first 8-10 weeks) with the following nutrients per head per day proved beneficial in preventing mastitis/ lowering milk SCC.

- Vitamin 53000 IU + Beta- carotene 300 mg
- Zinc-methionine (180-360 mg Zn, 360-720 mg methionine)
- Copper @ 20 ppmi.e. about 200 mg
- Vitamin E 1000 IU during dry period and 500 IU for lactating cows
- Selenium @ 3 mg during dry period and 6 mg during lactation

**2. *Cytokines*:** Cytokines include interferons, interleukins, colony stimulating factors (CSF), and a variety of other proteins that modulate the activity of immune cells and thus enhance the phagocytic cell functions in the udder. It has been shown that interferon treated cells exhibit significantly more phagocytosis and intracellular killing of *S. aureus*. Interleukins enhance the production of local antibodies and accelerate the involution process that will further promote resistance to mastitis during the dry period. Similarly, the granulocyte-macrophage CSF significantly increases the chemo tactic and bactericidal activities of mammary gland neutrophils.

**3. *Vaccination*:** The effective immunization against mastitis has been a goal of mastitis researchers for many years. But, the nature of disease creates a number of unique challenges for the production of successful immunity against mastitis. Commercially, few mastitis vaccines are currently available in developed world for immunization against mastitis caused by *Staphylococcus aureus* and *E. coli*. Several studies have evaluated these; the outcomes have been inconsistent and confusing to interpret. However, it is generally accepted that *S. aureus* vaccine have limited ability to prevent new infections and clinical mastitis cases. The best use of the vaccine is the reduction of chronic infections rather than prevention of new infections. The use of vaccine against coliforms mastitis has been considered efficacious even though the rate of IMI is not significantly reduced in vaccinated animals but because they significantly reduced the severity of clinical disease.

## Conclusion

Once mastitis is diagnosed the main challenge for the veterinarian or the producer is to treat the animals in such a way that it will not deteriorate and become an economic burden to the production system. Several therapeutic strategies like antibiotics, vaccines, bacteriocins, herbal therapy, immunotherapy, and nanoparticle technology have been evaluated for efficacy in treating mastitis, but no single technique was found to be effective in controlling or treating the disease due to the variable response of etiological agents to the therapeutic techniques.

## Suggested Readings

Bansal B K, Hamann J, Grabowski Nils Th and Singh K B. (2005a) Variation in the composition of selected milk fraction samples from healthy and mastitic quarters, and its significance for mastitis diagnosis. Journal of Dairy Research 72(2): 144-52.

Bansal B K and Gupta D K. (2009) Economic analysis of bovine mastitis in India and Punjab: A review. Indian Journal of Dairy Science 67:337-45.

Barkema H W, Schukken Y H and Zadoks R N. (2006) Invited Review: The role of cow, pathogen and treatment regimen in the therapeutic success of bovine Staphylococcus aureus mastitis. Journal of Dairy Science 89: 1877-95.

Constable P.D, Hinchcliff K.W, Donem S H and Gruenberg W. (2016): Veterinary Medicine: A textbook of the diseases of cattle, horses, sheep, pigs and goats. Chapter 20, Mastitis. Elsevier Health Sciences. 2113-2208.

De Oliveira A P, Watts J L, Salmon S A and Aarestrup F M. (2000. Antimicrobial susceptibility of Staphylococcus aureusisolated from bovine mastitis in Europe and the United States. Journal of Dairy Science 83: 855-62.

Radostits O M, Blood D C, Gay C C and Constable P D. (2007) Veterinary Medicine: Diseases of Cow, Buffalo, Horse, Sheep, Goat and Pig, 10thEdn. Saunders Elsevier Limited, Philadelphia, USA.

Steeve Giguere, John F. Prescott, Patricia M (2013)Antimicrobial Therapy in Veterinary Medicine 5thed.Wiley-Blackwell.

Viguier C, Arora S, Gilmartin N, Welbeck K and O'Kennedy R. (2009) Mastitis detection: current trends and future perspectives Trends in Biotechnology 27(8): 486-93.

# 8

# Animal Diseases on Farms Management Practices

***Vishal Mahajan***

*Animal Disease Research Centre, Guru Angad Dev Veterinary and Animal Sciences University, Ludhiana, Punjab*

## Abstract

*Livestock farms face significant threats from animal diseases, impacting animal health, productivity, and economic sustainability. Effective disease management and prevention strategies are imperative to mitigate outbreak risks. A proactive, collaborative approach involving farm personnel, veterinarians, and animal health authorities is crucial. Several prevalent animal diseases affect farms, including Haemorrhagic Septicemia (HS), Black Quarter, Listeriosis, Foot and Mouth Disease (FMD), Lumpy Skin Disease (LSD), Peste des Petits Ruminants (PPR), Sheep Pox, Blue Tongue, Swine Pox, Classical Swine Fever (CSF), and African Swine Fever (ASF).Prevention and management strategies vary for each disease but commonly include vaccination, early detection, diagnosis, monitoring, rapid response, and control measures. Diagnostic methods encompass postmortem examination, sample collection, culture, and molecular characterization. Vaccination is pivotal in disease prevention, with various vaccines available. Additionally, strict biosecurity measures, vector management, and government-authorized testing facilities are essential components of disease control. Overall, proactive disease management, encompassing vaccination, surveillance, biosecurity, and stakeholder collaboration, is essential for mitigating the impact of animal diseases on farm operations and ensuring livestock health and well-being.*

**Keywords:** Common diseases, Livestock Farms, Management, Precision Farming

Animal diseases on livestock farms can have significant impacts on animal health, farm productivity, and economic sustainability. Effective disease management and prevention strategies are crucial to minimize the risk of disease outbreaks and their consequences. Managing animal diseases requires a proactive and collaborative approach involving farm personnel, veterinarians, and animal health authorities. By implementing a combination of prevention, early detection, diagnosis, monitoring, rapid response and control measures, farms can effectively manage and mitigate the impact of diseases on animal health and farm operations. Outlined below are several prevalent animal diseases that can affect farms, along with prevention and management strategies.

## Haemorrhagic Septicemia (HS)

It is an acute infectious disease of cattle and buffaloes characterized by sudden onset, high fever, edematous swelling of subcutaneous tissues particularly under the neck, pneumonia and fatal septicemia. HS is highly infectious OIE enlisted disease caused by two specific serotypes of *Pasteurella multocida,* the Asian serotype B:2 and the African serotype E:2. It causes huge economic losses to dairy farmers of Asia and Africa due to high morbidity and case fatality. The outbreaks of HS are quite common in North region of the country

- Commonly encountered during and post rainy season but nowadays, reported throughout the year.
- The organism is normal commensal of nasopharynx and tonsils of livestock and under stress conditions, produces disease in animals.
- The disease is more common in buffalo than cattle. Animals of all ages are susceptible but disease is most common in 6 months to 2 years of age.
- Characterized by high fever, profuse salivation, respiratory symptoms, swelling under the neck and throat sounds and fatal septicemia; but typical swelling under neck is rarely reported nowadays.
- Diagnosed mainly on Post mortem lesions (froth in trachea, fibrinous deposit on lungs, marbling and adhesions of lungs to rib case, lungs severely consolidated giving it liver like consistency; all visceral organs exhibit petechial to ecchymotichemorrhages on serosal and mucosal surfaces).
- Sample required: nasal swab/ jugular blood of live animal, heart blood and lung sample of recently dead animal, or a bone marrow from a long bone of a carcass. The samples should be collected in nutrient broth.
- Confirmation of the disease on the basis of characteristic postmortem lesions, isolation and molecular characterization of the organism.
- Antibiotic treatment is effective if it is started very early, during the pyrexia stage. Drug of choice: enrofloxacin, gentamicin, ceftiofur.

Control is by vaccination of healthy animals with alum-precipitated vaccines (can be used in outbreaks) and oil adjuvant vaccine and revaccination should be done after every six months.

## Black-Quarter

Black quarter is an acute febrile disease affecting cattle. It leads to emphysematous swelling, typically in heavy muscles. The cause is *Clostridium chauvoei*, a gram-positive, spore-forming bacterium found in animal intestines and soil.The disease is more common in cattle aged 6 months to 2 years, with a 100% fatality rate. Occurs in summer and autumn, mostly in rapidly growing, well-fed cattle. Soil disturbance might trigger outbreaks. Transmission happens through contaminated feed, soil, or decomposed carcasses. The symptoms include sudden onset, high fever, painful muscle swelling, edema, and cracked, discolored skin. Swelling is usually in one limb, but can appear elsewhere too. Dark, frothy fluid with sour odor escapes when swelling is cut. Death occurs swiftly, within 12-36 hours.

- Diagnosis is based on timing, age, and necropsy.
- Culture is difficult. The cultural examination can be attempted by needle puncture or on swabs from wounds, but the organisms are very difficult to culture. The smears of affected tissues should be made particularly from the muscle tissues and heart blood. The samples of muscles should be taken immediately after death.
- Affected animals should be treated with large doses of penicillin 10000 IU/Kg body weight, starting with crystalline penicillin intravenously followed by long-acting preparations.
- During outbreak, isolation of affected animals and carcasses should be burnt or buried deep with lime. The skin of dead animals should not be removed.
- In endemic areas, control is by vaccination of healthy animals with alum-precipitated vaccines (can be used in outbreaks) and revaccination should be done yearly.

## Listeriosis

Listeriosis caused by *Listeria monocytogenes* is an infectious disease affecting wide range of animals including ruminants, monogastric animals and man. The disease occurs in three forms encephalitic, septicemic and abortions however, encephalitis is the most prevalent manifestation in sheep.

- In encephalitic form, nervous symptoms of circling, unilateral facial paralysis, unilateral blindness, dropping of ears and jaw. The infection results from trigeminal nerve infection consequent to abrasions of the buccal mucosa with feed or infection of tooth cavities.

Cerebrospinal fluid reveals higher concentration of total proteins with increase in globulins.

- Histopathologically, micro-abcesses and perivascular cuffing in the brain are pathognomonic lesions of disease.
- Sample required: Brain stem (Medulla oblongata, Pons and cerebellum).

Diagnosis can be made by characteristic clinical symptoms, histopathological findings isolation of organism, Immunohistochemistry and PCR.

- Drug of choice: Penicillin-G @ 44000 IU /kg body weight daily intramuscularly for 1-2 weeks.

**Foot and Mouth Disease (FMD)**

FMD is highly contagious disease enlisted in OIE list of notifiable diseases that infects cloven-hoofed animals *viz.* cattle, buffalo, sheep, goat, pig, camel and deer. The disease is caused by an aphthovirus (family Picornaviridae), which has seven major serotypes O, A, C, Asia 1 and Southern African Territories (SAT 1, SAT 2, SAT 3). Out of these serotypes (O, A, C, Asia 1) C strain has not been reported from India from last 30 years so this strain has removed from vaccine. It is probably the most important livestock disease in the world in terms of economic significance. Although FMD does not result in high mortality in adult animals, the disease has debilitating effects, including weight loss, decrease in milk production, and loss of draught power, resulting in a loss in productivity for a considerable time.

- In cattle, disease is characterized by fever, excessive salivation, lameness, formation of vesicles (fluid-filled blisters) and erosions in the mouth, nose, teats and feet. In young animals "Tiger heart" lesions on the myocardium may be seen.
- Sheep and goats are considered maintenance hosts and show mild clinical signs viz. fever, oral lesions and lameness.
- Pigs act as amplifying hosts and show more severe hoof lesions along with vesicles on the snout, however drooling of saliva may not be noticed.

- Sample collection: Vesicular epithelium from the lesions, whole blood, serum sample and esophageal-pharyngeal fluid.
- Laboratory diagnostic techniques include sandwich-ELISA, NSP-ELISA (Differentiation of vaccinated and infected animals) and PCR. Can also perform virus isolation.
- The symptomatic treatment includes antibiotics to check secondary bacterial infection, anti-inflammatory and antipyretic drugs. In addition, antiseptic mouth and teat wash can be given with potassium permagnate solution (1: 1000) or 2-5% povidine iodine solution. Besides, boroglycerine paste can be applied on mouth ulcers. The feet should be dipped in phenyl or 2% copper sulphate. In addition, provide easily chewable diet to the animals like dalia and lush green fodder.
- FMD prevention involves vaccinating animals with the trivalent oil adjuvant vaccine starting at the age of 4 months and subsequently, animals are vaccinated after every six months to maintain and boost their immunity.
- During an outbreak, steps to control FMD may include vaccination, surveillance, quarantine measures, establishment of control zones, strict biosecurity, reporting of confirmed cases, and hygienic measures.

## Lumpy Skin Disease (LSD)

Lumpy skin disease (LSD) is caused by lumpy skin disease virus (LSDV), a virus from the family Poxviridae, genus Capripoxvirus. Sheeppox virus and goatpox virus are the two other virus species in this genus. This virus is responsible for the development of characteristic skin nodules or lumps on the affected animals, primarily cattle, as well as water buffalo and other ruminants. These nodules can lead to discomfort, reduced milk production, and even secondary infections if not managed properly. The virus is mechanically transmitted through biting insects like mosquitoes and ticks. These insects acquire the virus from infected animals and then pass it on to healthy ones. Direct contact with an infected animal has a minor role in transmission. Infected bulls can shed the virus in semen, while skin nodules, scabs, and crusts contain high viral loads. The virus remains isolatable from these materials for up to 35 days and potentially longer. LSDV can also be found in blood, saliva, ocular and nasal discharges, and semen. The virus intermittently exists in the blood (viraemia) from around 7 to 21 days post-infection, typically in lower concentrations than in skin nodules. Viral shedding in semen might be extended.

Effective prevention and control of LSD are pivotal for safeguarding animal well-being, curtailing economic losses, and securing the livestock sector. The establishment of robust prevention measures and testing facilities is paramount.

- Vaccination: Immunization with heterologous (goatpox virus) and homologous vaccines is a primary preventive strategy for LSD. Young calves should be vaccinated at 3 to 4 months of age and revaccinated annually. Newly acquired animals should be vaccinated 28 days before integration into the herd. Pregnant and healthy cows/heifers can also be safely vaccinated. Full protection from the vaccine takes approximately three weeks to develop. During this period, animals may still encounter the field virus and display symptoms despite vaccination. In some cases, animals might already be incubating the virus during vaccination, leading to symptom manifestation within ten days post-vaccination.
- Biosecurity Practices: Rigorous biosecurity measures are crucial to impede the introduction and dissemination of the virus. Measures include controlled farm access, equipment disinfection, and limited interaction with animals from other farms.
- Vector Management: Effective control of insects like flies and ticks, which can transmit the virus, is essential. Use of insecticides, repellents, and environmental modifications can reduce vector populations. Isolation: Isolating newly acquired animals before their introduction to the herd prevents the introduction of potential virus carriers.
- Government of India, Department of Animal Husbandary and dairy has authorized college of Animal Biotechnology, Guru AngadDev Veterinary and Animal Sciences University for PCR/Real time PCR testing/screening of LSD in region (Chandigarh, Punjab, Ladakh, Jammu & Kashmir) for repeated incidences in the area confirmed by ICAR-NIHSAD, Bhopal.

**Peste des Petits Ruminants (PPR)**

PPR is highly contagious viral disease of domestic and wild small ruminants caused by *Moribilli-virus* belonging to family *Paramyxoviridae*and is clinically similar to rinderpest making differential diagnosis difficult. The country is now free from rinderpest, but unfortunately, PPR has become endemic in the country.

- Clinical signs exhibited include fever (105-107°F), ocular and nasal discharges, white cheesy deposits on the tongue and gums, labored breathing and occasional cough,feces are loose and watery that soil the posterior region of the affected animals.

- Post mortem lesions include inflammatory and necrotic lesions in the oral cavity and throughout the GI tract; “zebra stripes” of large intestine.
- Samples required include unclotted blood, serum, swabs of nasal and rectum, mediastinal and mesenteric lymph node, spleen, lungs, tonsils.
- Confirmation of disease can be done by sandwich ELISA (which is rapid and sensitive, and differentiates between PPR and rinderpest), virus isolation and PCR.
- There is no specific treatment, however, broad spectrum antibiotics to control secondary bacterial complications can be given along with supportive therapy.
- A live attenuated cell culture vaccine for PPR provides immunity for more than three years and booster immunization is not required. The vaccine is safe in animals older than 3 months. However, in endemic area annual vaccination is recommended.

### Sheep pox

A contagious disease of small ruminants caused by a sheep poxvirus classified in the genus *Capripoxvirus*of the family *Poxviridae*.

- Fever (106◦F), ocular and mucopurulent nasal discharge and difficult breathing; vesicle and pustule formation over the entire body surface mainly in the region of sparsely wooled area involving nostril, lip, ventral surface of tail, medial region of thigh, inguinal and udder region.
- Postmortem examination: Nodular lesion on the lung and whitish necrotic areas in kidneys. Histopathologically, there is eosinophilicintracytoplasmic inclusion bodies characteristic feature of sheep pox.
- Samples required: Skin biopsies, lymph nodes, lung lesion and serum sample.
- Diagnosis: History, Clinical signs, histopathological lesions and the confirmation of the disease by capripox diagnostic PCR.
- All diseased animals should be treated with broad-spectrum antibiotics to restrict secondary bacterial infections. Live attenuated vaccine prepared from the Romanian strain of SPV or Srinagar strain is being used for prophylaxis against sheep pox.

## Bluetongue

It is infectious, non-contagious disease of sheep and less commonly of cattle and goats characterized by catarrhal stomatitis, rhinitis, enteritis and lameness due to inflammation of coronary band and sensitive laminar of hooves.

- Fever (105-106°F) persist for few days, and then becomes normal.
- Reddening of buccal mucosa, excessive salivation, edema of lips and whole of face may be involved. Buccal mucosal hyperemic in early stages and become cyanotic later on. Formation of erosions in epithelium of mouth, lips, tongue and later on ulcer formation takes place ultimately necrosis, mucopurulent nasal discharge.
- The lameness is due to inflammation of coronary band (coronet). The lesions on the foot appear in some cases when buccal lesions start healing. Appearance of dark red or purple coloured band just above coronet is an important sign.
- Hemorrhages at the base of pulmonary artery are characteristic postmortem lesion.
- Diagnosis can be made by inoculation of blood in susceptible sheep or experimental mice, ELISA.
- Control is by vaccination with pentavalent inactivated vaccine containing BTV serotypes (BTV-1, 2, 10, 16, and 23) are commercially available (M/S Indian Immunologicals, Hyderabad).

## Swine Pox

Swinepox virus belongs to family *Poxviridae*and is characterized by typical poxvirus skin lesions in affected pigs and is generally seen in pig houses with poor sanitation. Infected swine are the main source of infection. Swinepox is most severe in young pigs (up to 4 months of age), where morbidity may approach 100 percent. Adults generally develop a mild, self-limiting form of the disease.The disease is transmitted by bite of louse, flies and insects as well as by direct contact. The disease can be seen concomitantly with swine fever outbreaks.

- Clinical signs include fever (105°F), typical pock lesions in the various stages of development ie. erythema, papules, vesicle and pustules on the face, ears, legs, and abdomen.
- Histopathological examination reveals large aggregates of eosinophilic inclusion in the cytoplasm characteristic feature of swine pox.

## Classical Swine Fever (CSF)

Classical swine fever (CSF), also known as hog cholera is a highly contagious viral disease of swine characterized by hemorrhages in internal organ in acute form and button ulcer in intestine in chronic form. CSF is caused by RNA virus belonging to the genus *Pestivirus*of the family *Flaviviridae*. It is the most important devastating disease responsible for very high morbidity and mortality, mummification of fetuses and abortions leading to huge economic losses to pig farmers. The disease is worldwide in distribution and has been reported frequently from various parts of India. Main route of infection is oro-nasal by direct or indirect contact with infected pig or feeding of inadequately cooked garbage.

- Clinical signs include fever (105°F), constipation followed by diarrhoea, gummed-up eyes, blotchy discoloration of the skin, abortion, still births and weak litters.
- Postmortem lesions include swollen and hemorrhagic lymph nodes, petechial to echhymotichemorrhages on kidney; splenic infarcts, button ulcers in cecum and colon are pathognomonic.
- Samples to be collected include tonsils, parotid glands, lymph nodes, spleen and kidneys.
- Diagnosis by clinical signs, post mortem findings.
- Laboratory diagnosis includes virus neutralization test and PCR.
- Broad-spectrum antibiotics can be given to check the secondary bacterial infections. Commercially available live tissue culture vaccines should be used for prevention of disease. Primary vaccine should be done at age of 2-3 months and then repeated after every 6 months.

## African Swine Fever

African swine fever (ASF) is one of the most contagious, emerging and deadly infectious disease in pigs. ASF is caused by large, double stranded DNA virus in the Asfarviridae family, genus Asfivirus. The disease spread very rapidly due to bite of ticks, improper hygiene and socioeconomic practices of animal handlers and movement of animals. It causes 100% mortality and non-availability of vaccines, which is a greatest concern to the pig industry around the globe.

- ASF infection cannot be detected based on the clinical signs and gross lesions because of the similarities classical swine fever, highly pathogenic porcine productive respiratory syndrome (PPRS) and salmonellosis.

- The spread of ASF can be prevented only by early detection and the strict application ofclassical disease control methods, including surveillance, epidemiological investigation, tracing of pigs, stamping out in infected stocks,quarantine, andman - animal movement control.
- In this current situation, effective bio-security measures are highly required for the proper containment of the diseases. The area covered under 1 km radius is declared as infected zone (IZ). An area of 10 km from infected premises is considered as surveillance zone (SZ) and beyond that is disease free zone (DFZ).
- Government of India, Department of Animal Husbandary and dairy has authorized college of Animal Biotechnology , Guru Angad Dev Veterinary and Animal Sciences University for Real time PCR screening of ASF in northern region (Punjab, Ladakh, Jammu & Kashmir, Chandigarh, Haryana, Himachal Pradesh, UP, NCT Delhi, Uttarakhand, Rajasthan) for repeated incidences in the area confirmed by ICAR-NIHSAD, Bhopal.

## Parasitic Diseases

### Fasciolosis

Fascioliosis caused by *Fasciola gigantica* in Punjab is very common parasitic disease. It is of economic importance not only in sheep or cattle but it may infect all domestic animals and wild animals may act as a source of infection for grazing sheep and cattle.

- Clinical signs include emaciation, loss of condition, anorexia, bottle jaw, diarrhoea, dyspnea, anemia, slight rise in temperature ($104^0$F) and serosanguinous nasal discharge.
- Samples to be collected include feces, serum and blood in EDTA from infected animals and tissue from all visceral organs from dead animals.
- Diagnosis is based on examination of fecal samples using sedimentation method revealing *Fasciola* eggs; and presence of intermediate host viz. snail (Lymnea) in the area there is high-rise of serum SGOT and SGPT enzymes.

## Amphistomiosis

Amphistomiosis is one of the most devastating disease of ruminants. Clinical disease is caused by immature flukes.The animals remain "carriers" or even at times suffer from outbreaks of the disease. Affected animals suffer from high morbidity and mortality.

- Clinical signs include emaciation, loss of condition, anorexia, bottle jaw, foetid diarrhoea, anaemia.
- Samples to be collected include feces, serum and blood in EDTA from infected animals.
- Diagnosis is based on finding immature flukes in faeces, examination of fecal samples using sedimentation method revealing typical amphistome eggs and presence of intermediate host viz. snails (*Indoplanorbis* spp.) in the area.

## Babesiosis

Bovine babesiosis is a febrile, tick-borne disease of cattle, caused by one or more protozoan parasites of the genus *Babesia*and generally characterized by extensive erythrocyticlysis leading to anemia, icterus, hemoglobinuria and death.

- Diagnosis is based on history of tick infestation (*Rhipicephalus (Boophilus) microplus)*, clinical signs such as fever and hemoglobinuria.
- Post-mortem findings: Marked jaundice, spleenomegaly, hepatomegaly, thick granular bile from gall bladder and urinary bladder filled with coffee colored urine.
- Confirmation by identification of pear-shaped bodies joined at an acute angle within the mature erythrocyte.
- Drug of choice is Diminazineaceturate (Berenil) @ 3-5 mg/kg BWt. deep intramuscularly

## Theileriosis

Bovine tropical theileriosis is a tick-transmitted protozoal disease of cattle caused by*Theileria annulata* characterized by high fever and lymphadenopathy. The disease causes high mortalities in breeds non-indigenous to the endemic areas, and is endemic in entire region.

- Diagnosis is based on history of tick infestation (*Hyalomma anatolicum anatolicum*), crossbred animals, clinical signs such as high fever and lymphadenopathy.
- Post-mortem findings: lymph nodes are edematous and hyperemic; punched necrotic ulcers in abomasums, marked jaundice.
- In the field, diagnosis is usually achieved by finding pleomorphic piroplasms (mainly rod shaped; however, round, oval, comma and ring-shaped forms also seen) in Giemsa-stained blood smears and schizont-infected cells in lymph node needle biopsy smears.
- Drug of choice is buparvaquone and halofuginone.

### Anaplasmosis

Anaplasmosis is an important disease of domestic animals caused by an obligate intraerythrocytic rickettsial parasite belonging to Genus *Anaplasma.* Disease is characterized by emaciation, anemia and jaundice. The affected animals show signs of fever anorexia and slightly enlarged lymph nodes. Disease is transmitted by ticks or by contaminated needles used for vaccination/treatment of animals.

- Post-mortem findings include severe jaundice, hepatomegaly and splenomegaly.
- Laboratory findings reveal small, dark red, round bodies present at the margin of the red cells in blood smears stained with Giemsa stain.
- Drug of choice includes high doses of oxytetracycline.

### Trypanosomosis

'Surra' is an acute, sub-acute or chronic disease of domestic animals caused by T*rypanosoma evansi* and characterized by fever, progressive emaciation, anemia, subcutaneous edema, nervous signs and death.

- Post-mortem findings includepetechiaehemorrhages and congestion on all visceral organs, spleenomegaly, and intestine filled with frank blood and ecchymotichaemorrhages on epicardium.
- Laboratory findings reveal trypanosomes in blood smears stained with Giemsa stain. There is slight decrease in haemoglobin.Morphologically Kinetoplast is sub-terminal in *T. evansi*. It has well developed undulating membrane, substantial free flagellum.
- Drug of choice: Quinpyramin Sulphate.

## Disease Testing of Farms for Infectious Diseases

Testing for infectious diseases is of paramount importance in farm management to ensure animal health, welfare, and productivity. Animals should undergo testing for the following diseases: Bovine brucellosis, Bovine Tuberculosis (TB) and Johne's disease (JD).

### Brucellosis

Brucellosis is quite common in Indian conditions and every case of abortion in the last trimester of pregnancy is viewed as that of brucellosis. *Brucella spp.* is facultative intracellular pathogens that have the ability to survive and multiply in phagocytes, and cause abortion in the domestic animals and undulant fever in the humans. Cattle are mainly affected with *B. abortus* and less commonly by *B. melitensis;* swine with *B. suis,* goats and sheep with *B. melitensis, B. ovis* causes epididymitis in ram.

This classification is mainly based on the differences in the pathogenicity and in host preference. *Brucella* strains may occur as either smooth or rough, expressing smooth LPS (S-LPS) or rough LPS (R-LPS) as major surface antigen. *B. abortus*, *B. suis* and *B. melitensis* carry a smooth LPS whereas *B. canis* and *B. ovis* possess rough LPS involved in the virulence of these bacteria. The bacterium possesses an unconventional non-endotoxic lipopolysaccharide that confers resistance to antimicrobial attacks and modulates the host immune response.

- The presumptive diagnosis can be made by identification of organisms in the stained smears from contaminated material using modified Ziehl-Neelson staining and confirmatory diagnosis depends on the isolation of Brucella from cervical mucus, uterine discharges, fetal stomach contents, placenta, supramammary and ileac lymph nodes.
- Rose Bengal Plate test (RBPT) is used for the early detection of Brucella specific agglutinins. The test is very sensitive especially in vaccinated animals. Positive samples should be retested by confirmatory test such as CFT or ELISA. Sometime non-specific reactions are caused by vaccination and occasionally by infection with other gram-negative bacteria such as *Yersinia* and *Salmonella.* As animals may be in the incubation stage of disease at the time of testing, a single negative result should not be taken as clear evidence of freedom from infection, and a second test should be carried out 30-60 days later or after 14 days of calving when serum antibody titre rises rapidly.

- *B. abortus* antigen, routinely used in the serological tests can detect *B. abortus*, *B. melitensis* and *B. suis* strains due to presence of smooth LPS, however, *B. canis* and *B. ovis* strains require specific test as they have rough LPS in their cell wall.
- Indirect ELISA is used for screening or as a supplemental test to the complement fixation test. The ELISA test has superior sensitivity over RBPT and reliably detects true negative results. OIE prescribed Indirect ELISA test for international trade.
- Competitive ELISA is most sensitive and specific test and used to distinguish the reactions caused by vaccination or infection.
- Several PCR protocols have been developed for identification of *Brucella abortus.* PCR based assays have been proved to be an important alternative rapid technique that overcome problems and disadvantages of currently used traditional methods.
- The *Brucella abortus* strain 19 vaccine is used for the prevention of brucellosis in cattle, specifically in calves and is administered to female calves within the age group of 4 to 8 months. This vaccination is given once in the lifetime of the calf to provide protection against brucellosis.

## Bovine Tuberculosis (TB)

Tuberculosis is an infectious, chronic, debilitating and granulomatous disease caused by acid-fast bacilli of the genus *Mycobacterium.* The disease affects all species of vertebrates and is characterized by progressive development of tubercles in the organs of most species. There are three types of tubercle bacilli *M. tuberculosis, M. bovis*, and *M. avium* in human, bovine, and avian species, respectively. These types differ in the cultural characteristics and pathogenicity, and may produce infection in other host species. *M. bovis* causes bovine tuberculosis and can cause progressive disease in most warm-blooded vertebrates, including man.

- Gross examination- (classic 'tuberculous' granulomas) and histology.
- Culturing the bacteria- culture usually taking long time up to 4-8 weeks.
- Acid-fast staining-bacterium is red while the other non-mycobacterium will be blue - The mycobacteria are acid fast. Organisms do not take up dyes of Gram stain as their cell wall is rich in lipids particularly mycolic acid. They are acid fast, as once cells take up dye, they are not easily decolourized even by acid alcohol. The mycobacteria are most closely

related to genera *Nocardia* and *Rhodococcus* and all three genera have similar cell wall type. Acid-fast organisms take red/pink stain whereas non-acid fast stain blue in colour.

- Single intradermal tuberculin test is standard method of diagnosis in live cattle in developing countries and is the prescribed test for international trade. It works on the principle of delayed-type hypersensitivity response. False negative results may occur in animals with poor immunity such as those in the early stages of infection, anergic cases in advanced disease, or old animals. Cattle that have recently calved may also have false negative results. TB positive cows go through a period of desensitization immediately before and after calving. In late pregnancy, fixed cell antibodies from skin come into general circulation and drain into colostrum, as a result dam may show false negative results for 4-6 weeks after parturition and calves which take the colostrum may show false positive results for up to 3 weeks. Besides, animals desensitized by tuberculin during preceding 8-60 days (tested for TB 8-60 days back) may show false negative results as the antibodies had already been used by early antigen. Besides, false positive reactions may occur due to sensitization to other *Mycobacteria* species such as human or avian TB, Johne's disease or other organisms like *Nocardia farcinicus*.
- Comparative Intradermal Test is used to differentiate infections caused by avian and mammalian mycobacteria. In this, both types of tuberculin are injected simultaneously 12 cm apart in neck area one above the other. Greater of the two reactions will indicate organism responsible for causing sensitization.
- ELISA or gamma interferon assay (γ-IFN) & PCR -ELISA and gamma interferon assays are valuable, with ESAT-6 and CFP-10 antigens improving bovine TB diagnosis. Polymerase chain reaction (PCR) offers rapid, sensitive DNA detection. In the live animals. Theγ- IFN assay test measures in vitro proliferation of stimulated T-cells from *M. bovis*infected animals on the basis of production of cytokine IFN-γ, which is predominantly released by T-cells after antigenic stimulation. Cytokine release assays, particularly the IFN-γ test, are being increasingly used internationally for the diagnosis of tuberculosis in animals due to the ready availability of commercial reagents.

## Paratuberculosis (Johne's disease)

Johne's disease is a chronic enteritis affecting ruminants, with Mycobacterium avium subspecies paratuberculosis (MAP) as the causative agent. The disease poses economic losses and links to human Crohn'sdisease. Although infection may occur at age of less than 30-days, but clinical disease usually occurs between 2 to 5 years of age. *MAP* bacteria are obligate pathogenic parasites of animals, and can multiply only inside an animal in the macrophages. The primary source of infection is infected animals. The entry of organism in the host mainly occurs via feco-oral route, such as through the ingestion of fecal contaminated milk or colostrum. Neonatal and juvenile animals are at the highest risk of acquiring the *MAP* infection. Young animals particularly neonates are most commonly infected due to their poorly developed immune systems.

- History: progressive emaciation, chronic intermittent diarrhea.
- Screening of dairy herds: Johnin test that works on the principle of delayed-type hypersensitivity response.
- Acid fast staining of fecal smear
- Advanced diagnostic tests: serum and milk ELISA, PCR.

## Conclusion

Prevention and control of animal diseases on farms involve a combination of biosecurity practices, vaccination, disease diagnosis, proper nutrition, sanitation, regular health monitoring, and quick response to outbreaks. Collaboration with local Veterinary authorities, Veterinary universities and relevant experts is essential to develop effective disease management plans tailored to the specific needs of the farm and the animals being raised.

## Suggested Readings

Coetzer, J. A. W., & Tustin, R. C. (2nd *edition*). Infectious Diseases of Livestock. Oxford University Press.Cape Town, 2004.

OIE. (2017.) Manual of Diagnostic Tests and Vaccines for Terrestrial Animals. World Organisation for Animal Health.

Radostits, O. M., Gay, C. C., Hinchcliff, K. W., & Constable, P. D. (11th edition). Veterinary Medicine: A Textbook of the Diseases of Cattle, Sheep, Pigs, andGoats. Elsevier.2017.

S. Sharma, V. Mahajan and K. S. Sandhu. (Ist edition). Handbook of Infectious Animal Diseases. Guru Angad Dev Veterinary and Animal Sciences University. 2011.

V. Mahajan, M.S. Bal, S. Sharma, G. Filia and A. Singh. (Ist edition). Colour Atlas and Diagnostic Guide of Farm Animal Diseases. Guru Angad Dev Veterinary and Animal Sciences University. 2016.

# 9

# Role of Farm Biosecurity in Curbing Antimicrobial Usage and Resistance in Animal Husbandry

***Pankaj Dhaka and Jasbir Singh Bedi***

*Centre for One Health, College of Veterinary Science, Guru Angad Dev Veterinary and Animal Sciences University, Ludhiana, Punjab*

## Abstract

*Farm biosecurity, encompassing a set of comprehensive preventive measures, holds paramount importance in the current scenario of animal husbandry. With intensive farming practices increasing infectious disease risks, biosecurity safeguards animal health and welfare, product quality, and responsible husbandry. The implementation of biosecurity measures yields benefits such as enhanced animal health, good product quality, prevention of zoonotic diseases, and effective antimicrobial stewardship.External biosecurity protocols encompass stringent access controls, quarantine procedures, waste management systems, personnel education, and visitor management, aiming to prevent disease incursion onto the farm. Internal biosecurity strategies prioritize farm and animal management, comprehensive cleaning and disinfection regimens, optimal nutrition practices, vaccination programs, disease surveillance, and early detection mechanisms to mitigate disease propagation within and beyond the farm boundaries. Additionally, internal biosecurity may involve proper ventilation systems, pest control measures, water quality management, and regular veterinary oversight to ensure comprehensive disease prevention and control.The interconnectedness of farm biosecurity and antimicrobial resistance lies in reducing disease transmission, decreasing the reliance on antimicrobials. The key challenges to adopt proper biosecurity measures in animal husbandry include resource constraints and cultural norms, emphasizing the need for technological, professionals and policies-oriented support.Ultimately, a well-implemented farm biosecurity system acts as a bridge, minimizing disease transmission and ensuring a sustainable future for both animal agriculture and human health.*

**Keywords:** Antimicrobial Resistance; Antimicrobial Usage;Dairy animals; Farm Biosecurity; One Health.

Intensive farming operations are particularly vulnerable to an increased risk of biohazards due to their densely populated livestock and close confinement. This increased animal density creates an environment where diseases can spread rapidly if not adequately managed. To mitigate these risks and safeguard the health and productivity of dairy herds, stringent farm biosecurity measures are essential. Farm biosecurity, a comprehensive framework of preventive measures and protocols, has emerged as a pivotal strategy in ensuring animal health and curbing the rise of antimicrobial resistance (AMR). By prioritizing biosecurity, dairy farmers can maintain a healthy and disease-free environment for their animals, ultimately ensuring the quality and safety of dairy products while promoting sustainable and responsible farming practices. In recent years, the interconnected challenges of animal health and AMR have prompted a re-evaluation of agricultural practices and disease management strategies.

## What is Farm Biosecurity?

Farm biosecurity refers to the set of practices and measures employed to prevent the introduction and spread of infectious diseases within animal production systems. It encompasses a wide array of strategies, ranging from physical barriers and hygiene protocols to monitoring and surveillance programs. The core principle of farm biosecurity is to mitigate the risk of disease incursions by minimizing the exposure of animals to pathogens, thereby preventing outbreaks and reducing the need for antimicrobial interventions. This strategic approach can be broadly categorized into 'external farm biosecurity' and 'internal farm biosecurity', each addressing distinct aspects of disease prevention within the farm environment.

## External Farm Biosecurity: Disease Prevention at the Gates

External farm biosecurity pertains to practices aimed at reducing the risk of introducing infectious diseases to a herd. It involves stringent management systems designed to prevent the entry of pathogens onto the farm premises. This is achieved through controlled access mechanisms that restrict the movement of personnel, vehicles, and equipment. By minimizing external disease sources, such as visitors and wildlife, farms can significantly reduce the likelihood of disease introduction. Quarantine protocols play a crucial role in this phase, isolating newly acquired animals to prevent potential disease transmission. External biosecurity is the first line of defence, ensuring that diseases do not infiltrate the farm from external sources.

## Internal Farm Biosecurity: Curbing Disease Spread Within Farm

Internal farm biosecurity encompasses management practices that influence animal interactions within the farm, with the goal of reducing or preventing disease spread among farm animals. Proper animal housing and hygiene practices are key components, creating an environment that minimizes stressors and disease susceptibility. In this context, the disease monitoring and surveillance are essential for early detection and swift response to potential outbreaks. Farm workers' training and education foster awareness of disease prevention and responsible antimicrobial use, reducing the risk of disease spread within the farm.

## The Significance of Farm Biosecurity

The implementation of farm biosecurity measures yields a multitude of benefits, underscoring its critical role in modern animal husbandry:

a) *Enhanced Animal Health and Productivity:* Effective farm biosecurity measures result in healthier animals less prone to infectious diseases. This, in turn, boosts farm productivity and reduces healthcare-related costs, contributing to improved economic viability.

b) *Animal Welfare and Product Quality*: The adoption of robust biosecurity practices is linked to superior animal welfare and high-quality animal products. Animals reared in healthier environments yield better quality products for consumers.

c) *Zoonotic Disease Prevention:* Many animal diseases can transmit to humans as zoonotic infections, such as brucellosis and bovine tuberculosis. Proper farm biosecurity implementation, coupled with worker hygienic practices, acts as a barrier, preventing the transmission of these diseases to farmers and the public.

d) *Antimicrobial Stewardship:* A significant association exists between farm biosecurity and antimicrobial usage (AMU). Implementing biosecurity measures reduces disease incidence, subsequently lowering the need for antimicrobial treatments. This reduction in AMU contributes to curbing AMR in the food chain and the environment.

The outline of various external and internal biosecurity factors in dairy farm are highlighted in figure 1.

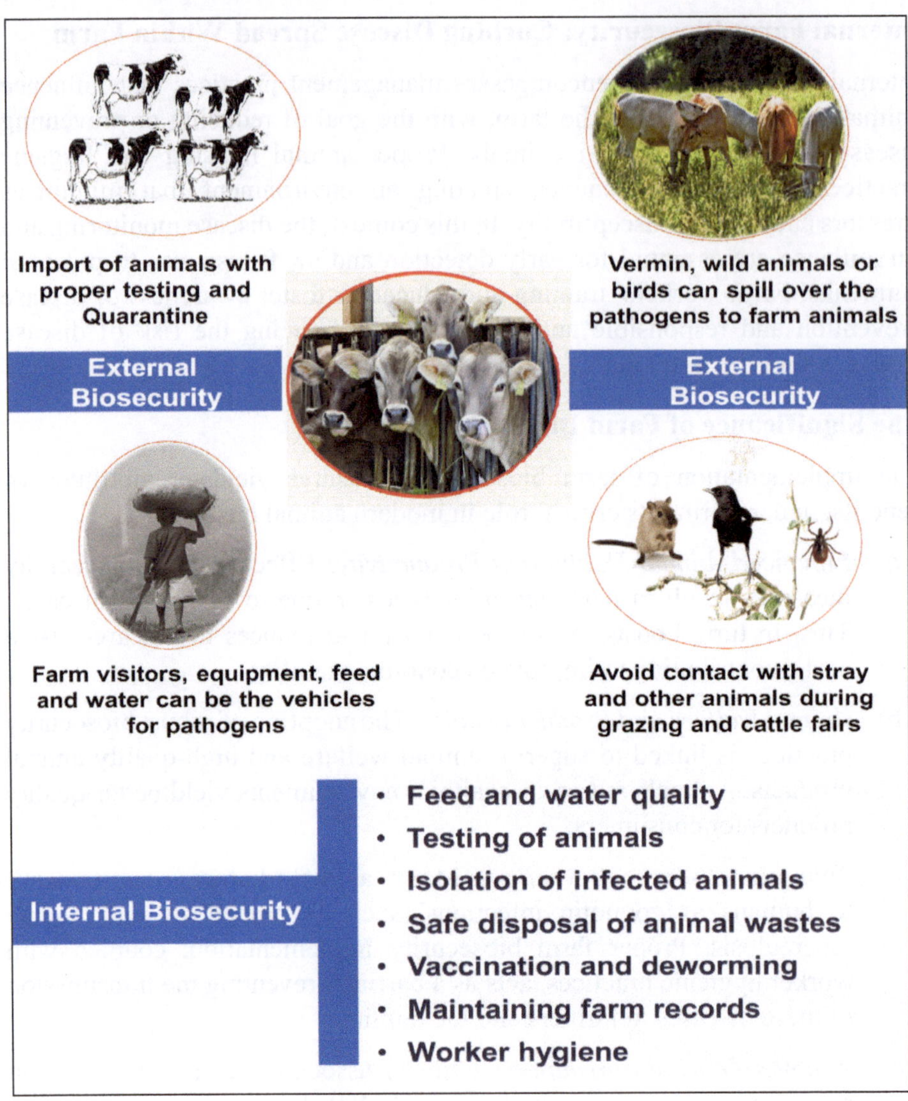


**Figure 1:** An illustration of various external and internal biosecurity factors in dairy farm.

## Factors Affecting AMU at Farm Level

Antimicrobial resistance is a growing global concern with serious implications for human and animal health. In the realm of animal husbandry, the misuse and overuse of antimicrobial agents have been identified as major drivers of AMR development. To effectively address this challenge, it is essential to explore the factors that contribute to the excessive use of antimicrobials and understand how farm biosecurity can play a pivotal role in mitigating their usage. This section explores the multifaceted factors influencing AMU in animal production systems and elucidates the critical role of farm biosecurity in addressing this issue.

a) ***Intensive farming practices and disease spread:*** Intensive farming practices, characterized by high stocking densities and close confinement of animals, create an environment conducive to disease transmission. Overcrowded and unsanitary conditions provide pathogens with ample opportunities to proliferate, leading to the rapid spread of infections. To combat the resultant disease outbreaks, farmers often resort to the prophylactic use of antimicrobial agents. This practice, while providing short-term relief, perpetuates a cycle of antimicrobial dependence and fosters the emergence of resistant pathogens.

b) ***Lack of disease surveillance and early detection:*** Inadequate disease surveillance and early detection mechanisms exacerbate the AMU problem. Without proper monitoring, farmers may not promptly identify the presence of pathogens within their herds or flocks. Consequently, infections can spread unchecked, necessitating aggressive antimicrobial interventions as a last resort. Farm biosecurity addresses this challenge by emphasizing routine health checks, diagnostic testing, and rapid response protocols. By swiftly identifying and isolating affected animals, biosecurity measures can curb the need for widespread antimicrobial treatments.

c) ***Suboptimal nutrition and immune function:*** Animals kept in suboptimal conditions are more susceptible to infections due to weakened immune systems. Malnutrition, inadequate access to clean water, and poor ventilation compromise an animal's ability to mount an effective immune response against pathogens. To counteract the resulting health issues, antimicrobial agents are frequently used to prevent or treat infections. Farm biosecurity, however, focuses on creating optimal conditions for animal welfare, including proper nutrition and housing. By strengthening immune function, biosecurity measures minimize the need for antimicrobial interventions.

d) ***Lack of knowledge and awareness:*** Limited knowledge about disease preventive aspects and the consequences of antimicrobial misuse can contribute to their inappropriate use. Some farmers may be unaware of alternative disease prevention methods or may underestimate the risks associated with AMR. Farm biosecurity interventions encompass educational initiatives that promote understanding and adoption of preventive measures. Training programs and information dissemination empower farmers with the tools to make informed decisions that reduce their reliance on antimicrobial treatments.

## How Farm Biosecurity can Play Role in Curbing AMU!

The health of animals within agricultural systems is vulnerable to a spectrum of challenges, including infectious diseases caused by bacteria, viruses, parasites, and fungi. These diseases not only result in significant economic losses due to decreased productivity and increased mortality but also contribute to the rising threat of AMR. The extensive use of antimicrobial agents in animal husbandry to control infections has led to the emergence of resistant pathogens, diminishing the effectiveness of these crucial drugs in both animals and humans.

The intricate connection between farm biosecurity and AMR is rooted in the overuse and misuse of antimicrobials in animal production. In environments with poor biosecurity measures, diseases can spread rapidly, necessitating the frequent application of antimicrobial agents to control outbreaks. This persistent use of antimicrobials contributes to the selection and proliferation of drug-resistant pathogens. By reducing disease transmission through strict biosecurity protocols, the reliance on antimicrobial treatments diminishes, decreasing the opportunities for resistant pathogens to emerge and spread.

Farm biosecurity offers a comprehensive approach to tackling the factors that drive AMU. These measures include controlled access of personnel, vehicles, and equipment to prevent the introduction of pathogens. Quarantine procedures isolate new animals to ensure they are disease-free before integration. Proper waste management and pest control mitigate the risk of disease transmission via vectors.

Biosecurity protocols also emphasize the importance of vaccination. Targeted vaccination programs provide animals with immunity against specific pathogens, reducing the likelihood of infections and the subsequent need for antimicrobial intervention. Additionally, biosecurity measures promote overall animal health through improved nutrition, housing, and hygiene, strengthening immune responses and diminishing susceptibility to diseases.

Farm biosecurity interventions offer a more sustainable and cost-effective approach. By focusing on disease prevention, biosecurity measures reduce the economic burden associated with disease outbreaks and subsequent treatments. Additionally, ethical considerations play a role, as responsible animal husbandry entails minimizing suffering and ensuring the well-being of animals under human care.

Some of the key components of external and internal farm biosecurity and their impact on curbing AMU.

### External Biosecurity Parameters

1) ***Controlled access:*** Limits the introduction of pathogens to the farm, reducing the risk of disease outbreaks that would require antimicrobial interventions.
2) ***Quarantine protocols*:** Isolation of new animals prevents the spread of potential diseases, minimizing the need for antimicrobial treatment.
3) ***Proper waste management*:** Reduces disease vectors and environmental contamination, lowering the likelihood of infections and the demand for antimicrobial use.
4) ***Biosecurity training and awareness*:** Educates farm personnel about biosecurity measures, leading to better disease prevention practices and decreased reliance on antimicrobials.
5) ***Farm design and layout*:** Proper layout prevents cross-contamination between different animal groups, reducing the need for widespread antimicrobial treatments.
6) ***Animal source selection*:** Careful selection of disease-free animals reduces the introduction of pathogens, minimizing disease occurrences and antimicrobial use.
7) ***Control of visitors and vendors*:** Limits external exposure to the farm, decreasing the risk of disease transmission and lowering the need for antimicrobials.
8) ***Biosecurity audits and certifications*:** Regular audits ensure compliance with biosecurity protocols, leading to better disease prevention and reduced antimicrobial use.
9) ***Wildlife and pest control:*** Minimizes potential carriers of diseases, reducing the need for antimicrobial interventions to treat resulting infections.
10) ***Water and feed quality control*:** Ensures clean water and uncontaminated feed, supporting animal health and reducing the need for antimicrobial treatments.

## Internal Biosecurity Parameters

1) ***Vaccination programs***: Targeted vaccination reduces the incidence of diseases, decreasing the need for antimicrobial use in treating infections.
2) ***Animal housing and hygiene***: Clean and well-maintained housing promotes animal health, minimizing stress and lowering susceptibility to infections, reducing AMU.
3) ***Disease surveillance and monitoring:*** Early detection and rapid response to diseases prevent their spread, reducing the severity of outbreaks and the necessity for antimicrobial treatments.
4) ***Health and welfare management***: Focusing on animal well-being strengthens immune systems, decreasing vulnerability to infections and subsequently the use of antimicrobials.
5) ***Proper nutritional practices***: Providing balanced nutrition supports strong immune function, reducing the need for antimicrobial treatments in response to malnutrition-related health issues.
6) ***Animal density and grouping***: Proper spacing and grouping prevent overcrowding and stress, reducing the likelihood of disease outbreaks and associated antimicrobial use.
7) ***Veterinary care and expertise***: Regular veterinary check-ups and intervention strategies minimize disease incidence, curbing the need for antimicrobial treatments.
8) ***Pathogen testing and management***: Regular testing identifies potential threats, enabling swift management to prevent disease outbreaks and antimicrobial use.
9) ***Record keeping and traceability***: Accurate records facilitate disease tracking and management, enabling targeted interventions and reducing the overall need for antimicrobials.
10) ***Biosecurity training for farm staff***: Educated staff adhere to better disease prevention practices, leading to fewer infections and lower AMU.

These parameters within both external and internal biosecurity play crucial roles in reducing the dependence on antimicrobial agents in animal husbandry. By effectively preventing and managing diseases, these measures contribute to the broader effort to combat AMR.

## Challenges and Implementation Hurdles

While the concept of farm biosecurity holds promise, its successful implementation is not without challenges. In many regions, limited resources and awareness hinder the adoption of biosecurity practices. Smaller, resource-constrained farms may struggle to invest in necessary infrastructure and training. Additionally, changing ingrained practices requires a shift in mindset and cultural norms. Governments and international organizations play a crucial role in overcoming these challenges by providing incentives, technical support, and regulations that encourage the adoption of biosecurity measures.

## A Call for a One Health Approach

The concept of One Health underscores the interconnectedness of human, animal, and environmental health. This approach is especially relevant when discussing farm biosecurity and AMR. Pathogens can cross the species barrier, affecting both animals and humans. Collaborative efforts among veterinarians, medical professionals, researchers, policymakers, and environmental experts are essential to comprehensively address these challenges. For example, veterinarians can provide insights into animal health, medical professionals can monitor human health impacts, and environmental scientists can track disease vectors. By pooling knowledge and resources, a more holistic and effective approach to farm biosecurity can be achieved. A well-implemented farm biosecurity system can serve as a critical bridge in this collaboration, helping to minimize disease transmission at the animal-human interface and subsequently reducing the pressure on AMU.

## Future Directions and Recommendations

The path forward involves a combination of innovative research, policy support, and ongoing collaboration. Researchers can explore new biosecurity technologies, such as sensor-based disease monitoring systems and precision vaccination approaches. Policymakers need to create an enabling environment by establishing clear guidelines, offering incentives for biosecurity adoption, and penalizing inappropriate antimicrobial use. International cooperation is crucial for sharing best practices and surveillance data, as diseases and resistance know no borders.

## Conclusion

In the face of the growing threat of AMR, farm biosecurity emerges as a beacon of hope for sustainable animal husbandry practices. By addressing the root causes of disease and minimizing the need for antimicrobials, biosecurity measures not only protect animal health but also safeguard human health and global food security. The One Health approach underscores the necessity of collaborative efforts that transcend traditional disciplinary boundaries. As we navigate the complex landscape of AMR, the role of farm biosecurity shines as a critical tool for ensuring the well-being of animals, humans, and the planet.

## Suggested Readings

Biosecurity- A Practical Approach. PennState Extension. (Weblink: https://extension.psu.edu/biosecurity-a-practical-approach)

Biosecurity and Biosafety Manual for Bovines. Government of India, Ministry of Agriculture & Farmers Welfare, Department of Animal Husbandry, Dairying & Fisheries (Weblink: https://www.dahd.nic.in/sites/default/filess/Biosecurity%20and%20biosafety%20manual%20for%20Bovines.pdf)

Dhaka, P., Bedi, J.S., Deepthi, V., Kaur, S., Singh, B.B., and Aulakh, R.S. 2021. 'Awareness Guide on Dairy Farm Biosecurity' [ISBN No. 978-93-5473-823-4]. (Weblink: https://www.researchgate.net/publication/358119581_Awareness_Guide_on_Dairy_Farm_Biosecurity)

Dhaka, P., Chantziaras, I., Vijay, D., Bedi, J.S., Makovska, I., Biebaut, E. and Dewulf, J., 2023. Can Improved Farm Biosecurity Reduce the Need for Antimicrobials in Food Animals? A Scoping Review. Antibiotics, 12(5), p.893.

Farm Worker Health and Hygiene Basic Rules. PennState Extension. 2019. (Weblink: https://extension.psu.edu/farm-worker-health-and-hygiene-basic-rules)

Renault, V., Humblet, M.F., Pham, P.N. and Saegerman, C., 2021. Biosecurity at Cattle Farms: Strengths, Weaknesses, Opportunities and Threats. Pathogens, 10(10), p.1315.

Thukral, H., Dhaka, P., Bedi. J.S., and Aulakh, R.S. Biosecurity: A Frontline Defence for Infectious Diseases on Dairy Farms. International Animal Health Journal, 2020, 7(3):50-54

World Organisation for Animal Health. How to Implement Farm Biosecurity: The Role of Government and Private Sector (Weblink: https://www.oie.int/fileadmin/Home/eng/Publications_%26_Documentation/docs/pdf/TT/2017_ASI1_Windsor.pdf)

World Organisation for Animal Health. Investing in biosecurity: a key step to curb the spread of animal diseases (Weblink:https://www.oie.int/en/for-the-media/press-releases/detail/article/investing-in-biosecurity-a-key-step-to-curb-the-spread-of-animal-diseases/)

# 10

# Breed Improvement for Enhancing Productivity of Dairy Animals in District Muzaffarnagar (UP): An Attempt

***Pawan Singh***

*Livestock Production Management ICAR – National Dairy Research Institute, Karnal, Haryana*

**Abstract**

*The ICAR-NDRI, Karnal is running a Kisan Seva Kendra at village Lalukheri of district Muzaffarnagar (UP) to cater the requirement of farmers for frozen semen doses, crops seed and mineral mixture. The centre has organised 35 meetings for farmers awareness for adopting scientific techniques/practices for dairy husbandry and animal health checkup camps in 25 villages. The Ministry of Fisheries, Animal Husbandry and Dairying has sanctioned Rs. 8.5 crores to NDRI to expand the present services of the centre in 100 villages of district Muzaffarnagar. Under the project, the farmers will be provided artificial insemination services at their door steps with superior quality Murrah buffalo and cow bulls semen for improving milk production potential of local breed, and the quality mineral mixture to feed their cows and buffaloes for improving their reproduction and production.*

**Keywords:** Breed improvement, Dairy animals, Productivity, Prcision Farming

ICAR-NDRI, Karnal is running a Kisan Seva Kendra at village Lalukheri of district Muzaffarnagar (UP) to cater the requirement of the farmers for frozen semen doses, crops seed and mineral mixture of villages around the center. This centre was established in year 2005; it started fully functioning in 2015. This centre is providing service to the farmers in ~25 villages around the centre. It provides frozen semen doses of high genetic merit bulls with the aim for making improvement in genetic potential for higher milk production of dairy animals of farmers in villages around the centre. The centre is also making available mineral mixture for improving fertility of dairy animals and also making available fodder crop seed to the farmers for growing quality fodder for their dairy animals. Kisan gosthis and farmers awareness camps are also being organized to increase farmers' awareness regarding benefits of rearing high producing dairy animals and feeding them balance ration for improving their production and reproduction performance.

Since 2015, center has organised ~35 meetings for farmers awareness for adopting scientific techniques/practicesfor dairy husbandry and animal health checkup camps in ~25 villages for improving production and fertility of dairy animals. The maximum numbers of progenies so far, through the use of frozen semen doses from the centre, have been produced of dairy cows and buffaloes in the village- Bhorakhurd (300), Sonjanikheri (440), Alipur (300), Sotta (250) and Sallakheri (250), total 1540 calves.

In this region, the average peak milk yield of a buffalo is ~ 8-10 litres per day i.e. the maximum milk produced on single day during the entire lactation. This has now gone to ~15 lits of milk in the progenies born of these animals with the use of high genetic merit bulls' frozen semen for artificial insemination. There are ~25 buffaloes in Bhorakhurd village alone produced ~15 litres of peak milk yield; whereas the milk yield of their dams was only ~8-10 litres. It means there is ~3-5 litres increase in milk yield of females born due the use of semen of high genetic merit buffalo bulls. The trend is same in other villages also where the females born with the semen of high genetic merit bulls was used for inseminating females. Also the farmers in this village have started use of mineral mixture to feed their animals which is making improvement in fertility of their dairy animals. Similar improvement in milk yield and fertility of dairy animals in other villages is also being observed. After seeing the progress in these villages in improvement of breed and in milk yield of animals had borne with inputs interms of frozen semen of high genetic merit bulls from best institutions like NDRI, Karnal; CIRB, Hisar and HLDB, Hisar, and mineral mixture from Govt institution. Now seeing the progress, in surrounding villages of NDRI Farmers Service Center at Lalukheri, in improvement of milk yield and fertility of dairy animals in the nearby villages; The Ministry of Fisheries, Animal Husbandry and Dairying has sanctioned Rs. 8.5 crores to NDRI to expands the present services of the centre in 100 villages of district Muzaffarnagar. Under the project, the farmers will be provided artificial insemination services at their door steps for that 35 inseminators have been recruited. The frozen semen doses of Murrah buffalo bull will be procured from the well-known stations having superior quality Murrah buffalo bulls in the country. The cow bulls semen doses will be procured from NDRI, karnal for improving milk production potential of local breed. Farmers are also being provided quality mineral mixture to feed their cows and buffaloes for improving their reproduction and production. Kisan gosthies are also being organised for making the farmers aware about the scientific rearing of dairy animals like balance ration formulation, use of semen of high quality bulls for AI in their animals, control of parasite of their animals etc.

General problems are faced in implementation such projects in the fields are listed below:

- **Non-availability of AI services to the farmers- timely and effectively**
- **Non-availability of liquid nitrogen supply to inseminators**
- **Lack of availability of AI servicesat farmers' door step-** Farmers do not get AI services as and when required at their doorsteps.
- **Lack of awareness among the farmers for importance of quality bull's semen** – they only go for AI of their animals without considering genetic merit of bulls.
- **Non-availability of such semen to farmers-** they have to depend on private inseminators, whatever bull's semen they/AI workers have farmer has to go for it, he has no choice before him.
- **Lack of availability of liquid nitrogen to the inseminators-** there is no effective system in place for AI implementation including availability of liquid nitrogen in the field.
- **Deficiency of trained/skill inseminators**– There is deficiency of skilled AI workers in the field for implementation of AI in dairy animals.

## References

Oltenacu, P. A., & Broom, D. M. (2010). The impact of genetic selection for increased milk yield on the welfare of dairy cows. Animal welfare, 19(S1), 39-49.

Singh, P., Mukesh, M., & Kumar, S. (2022). Artificial insemination: scope and challenges for indian dairy sector. In Advances in Animal Experimentation and Modeling (pp. 359-364). Academic Press.

Tomar, D. S., Lathwal, S. S., Singh, P., & Devi, I. (2023). Evaluation of productive and reproductive performance of dairy animals in district Muzaffarnagar of Uttar Pradesh.

# Index